EAT REAL FOOD AND LOVE IT:

6 STEPS TO HELP YOU CRAVE HEALTHY EATING

EAT REAL FOOD AND LOVE IT:

6 STEPS TO HELP YOU CRAVE HEALTHY EATING

Kari McCloskey MBA, RD

Copyright © 2022 by Kari McCloskey MBA, RD.

Library of Congress Control Number:		2022913203
ISBN:	Hardcover	978-1-6698-2666-8
	Softcover	978-1-6698-2665-1
	eBook	978-1-6698-2664-4

All rights reserved. No part of this book may be reproduced or transmitted in any form or by any means, electronic or mechanical, including photocopying, recording, or by any information storage and retrieval system, without permission in writing from the copyright owner.

Any people depicted in stock imagery provided by Getty Images are models, and such images are being used for illustrative purposes only. Certain stock imagery © Getty Images.

Print information available on the last page.

Rev. date: 11/09/2022

To order additional copies of this book, contact:
Xlibris
844-714-8691
www.Xlibris.com
Orders@Xlibris.com
843124

Contents

Dedication ix
Preface xi
Foreword xv
Acknowledgments xvii
Introduction xix

STEP 1

Chapter 1 Notice Your Current Patterns of Eating 1
Chapter 2 Notice What Nature's Foods Do for You 5
Chapter 3 Notice the Ingredients in Synthetic Foods 20
Chapter 4 Notice the Findings from Epigenetics and
             Nutrigenomics 27
Chapter 5 Notice Summary, Recommendations, and Action
             Steps 31

STEP 2

Chapter 6 Analyze by Learning a Food's Background 39
Chapter 7 Analyze the Quality of Wheat 46
Chapter 8 Analyze Meat 52
Chapter 9 Analyze Flavor Ingredients 56
Chapter 10 Analyze Sweeteners 66
Chapter 11 Analyze Food Advertising 71
Chapter 12 Analyze Produce 73
Chapter 13 Analyze Summary, Recommendations, and
             Action Steps 75

STEP 3

Chapter 14	Train Journey	89
Chapter 15	Train New Memories	92
Chapter 16	Train Your Brain to Retrain	98
Chapter 17	Train Your Habits	102
Chapter 18	Train Your Taste Buds	108
Chapter 19	Train Your Gut	112
Chapter 20	Train Yourself to Undo Stress	117
Chapter 21	Train Summary, Recommendations, and Action Steps	121

STEP 4

Chapter 22	Unite Your Foods to Work for You	133
Chapter 23	Unite Activity with Eating to Run Your Metabolism	138
Chapter 24	Unite Water with the Right Macros	148
Chapter 25	Unite the Right Amount of Sodium	161
Chapter 26	Unite Your Eating in a Plan	165
Chapter 27	Unite Movement with Eating	175
Chapter 28	Unite Movement and Eating with Meditation	184
Chapter 29	Unite Summary, Recommendations, and Action Steps	193

STEP 5

Chapter 30	Renew your Relationship with Food	199
Chapter 31	Renew Your Natural Opiates	202
Chapter 32	Renew Your Food Relationship, if Needed	207
Chapter 33	Renew Support	212
Chapter 34	Renew Your Reasons for Eating and Drinking	214
Chapter 35	Renew Your Readiness	216
Chapter 36	Renew Summary, Recommendations, and Action Steps	221

PART 6

Chapter 37 Enjoy Incentives 229
Chapter 38 Enjoy Small Steps with Age..233
Chapter 39 Enjoy Sharing..235
Chapter 40 Enjoy Summary, Recommendations, and Action
            Steps 238

References 245

Dedication

I'd like to dedicate this book to my Maker, the Creator of this beautiful world, who made all living things, including humans and plants. And to all the loves of my life—Roger, Victoria, Brett, Briana, Garrett, Marcus, Sophia, Sunny, Emerson, Kai, Levi, Josephine, and Dove—who all inspire me to be healthy so I can be a better person.

Preface

After seeing thousands of clients as an outpatient, hospital-based registered dietitian, I started to understand what drives so many people to be overweight and unhealthy. Ironically, everyone wants to enhance the quality of his or her life. No one intentionally decides that it's time to be stricken with a lifestyle disease or become obese. All people want to have life spans as long as, or longer than, their parents, grandparents, or great-grandparents. They also want to ensure the survival of the next generation. Yet the food and beverages they consume are causing their health and their children's health to deteriorate prematurely. The problem is simple: my clients' palates are conditioned to crave unhealthy food. However, the solution for better health and longevity is much more complicated: they need to *want* to eat what's good for them.

Eat Real Food and Love It attempts to assist you in making a paradigm shift from eating to please your brain to reclaiming the desire to consume what nature produces. Studies show there is an axis between your gut (digestive tract) and brain; [114] therefore, nourishing your gut will help your brain think better. If you want to get and stay healthy but find yourself craving foods and beverages that cause weight gain or affect your health negatively, know *you can learn how to crave what's good for you. You are designed to consume nature's foods and beverages. Your body knows how to do it.*

With all the advancements of modern technology and medicine, nothing can yet match the complex healing effects of Mother Nature. The foods that strengthen your mind and build your body physically, intellectually, emotionally, and spiritually are real foods from nature. Nature's foods give your body and mind the best building materials possible to help move you through life. I've always been fascinated by how the body works, and I hope this book will help to inspire you to find out how your unique body functions and discover tools you can use to take your health to the next level.

Because I have seen the devastating health effects of those who have developed a taste for commercially packaged, on-the-go foods and drinks, I want to help people shift their palates. The foods that have caused my clients to become ill are full of massive amounts of sugar, fat, salt, artificial ingredients, and preservatives. Yet these are the foods I used to indulge in. But now when people ask me, "Don't you just want a juicy steak or a doughnut once in a while?" or when I walk through a convenience store to grab something to eat and pass by the shelves of candy, cookies, and chips, I can honestly say, "I *don't want* those foods."

Why don't I crave processed foods today? I ate them years ago and loved them. I grew up in the Midwest on a steady diet of meat, burgers, pot pies, canned and frozen foods, candy, pies, doughnuts, juice, and soda (or "pop," if you're from the Midwest like me). I indulged at every fast-food restaurant and even worked at one as a teen.

As I look back at what I ate then compared it to how I eat now, I'm glad I changed. I used to consume foods and beverages full of chemicals I thought I needed to get me through the day. Those chemicals, however, were causing my moods to swing and my health to deteriorate. But today I don't eat the unhealthy foods I used to—not because I can't eat them but because I don't enjoy them. I now choose, for the most part, whole foods as close to the vine as possible. I eat predominantly a plant-based diet full of fresh fruit, whole grains, legumes, an abundance of raw and cooked vegetables, nuts, seeds, and occasionally wild seafood. And I enjoy their taste! I also like to cook healthy foods for others. Being both a mother and a "Nina" (my grandma name), I love to spend time in the kitchen, creating savory dishes out of plant foods. I also occasionally cook the highest-quality grass-fed, organic meats I can find for the meat eaters in my family. I stay away from factory-farmed and processed meats. (I'm not against people eating a small amount of meat a couple of times a week, but I personally don't eat it. One visit to a slaughterhouse while I was going through dietetics school years ago killed my desire to ever eat meat again.) I do like sweets, so I enjoy dark chocolate and low-sugar or fresh-fruit desserts.

The need for change was a personal journey to feel happier, combat depression, and be healthier. Now that I'm in my fifties, eating well helps me run around with my grandkids; be energetic, athletic, healthy, lean, and for the most part, happy. I now *crave* plant foods, which give me clarity and energy. I am actually drawn to eating vegetables because they *taste* good. This was a learned practice because I didn't discover vegetables until I was well into adulthood. Several years after I began replacing packaged processed foods with healthier plant-based foods, I had an epiphany: I was heading back to the way of eating my body was designed for, back to nature, the origin of how I was meant to eat. I was able to get there, and I want you to get there too.

My friend asked me one day, "How did you go from being a junk food addict to a health food champion?" Because I feel so much better now that I eat healthily, I want to share with you the process that worked for me and now works for my clients. My eating preferences have changed radically from how I used to eat, and I'm not alone. *I changed my brain so it enjoys and loves the taste of healthy foods. Others have also done it, and so can you.*

Foreword

As a physician, I am always on the lookout for real and practical solutions for my patients. Some of the biggest challenges my patients face are healthy eating and weight management. Many of my patients express a desire to lose weight, and be "healthier", and most have an understanding that a healthy diet is the first step towards achieving those goals. Unfortunately, there are a number of challenges and obstacles that prevent many from achieving their goals of healthier eating and improved health on a lifelong basis.

Therefore, I was very happy to discover EAT REAL FOOD AND LOVE IT: 6 STEPS TO HELP YOU CRAVE HEALTHY EATING. I believe this book fills the gaps that many of my patients struggle to overcome, and lays out a practical and sustainable approach to healthy eating and improved health.

I love Kari's 6 step approach! Although we may all want a quick fix to our dieting challenges, quick fixes are at best short-lived, and sometimes downright dangerous. Instead, Kari has laid out a very approachable and sustainable stepwise approach to health. I love how she begins by simply *Noticing*. Most of us have our usual routines and don't even notice our usual patterns of eating or the ingredients of our usual foods.

Kari next invites us to *Analyze* our diets and the modern industrial food industry. I was fascinated to read Kari's laying bare the history of the modern food industry, and the many ways that mass-produced foods are designed to appeal to and exploit our senses, yet ultimately undermine good health. Truly a wakeup call for us all to analyze our current eating patterns, and make more informed choices for better health.

Many of my patients are seeking a harmonious balance of diet and exercise, but don't know quite how to get there. Kari has done a very nice job of *Uniting* a healthy diet with exercise, water intake, eating plans, and even meditation into a cohesive whole-life approach to health.

Finally, I love how Kari describes *Renewing* and *Enjoying* as the final steps of a sustainable approach to healthy eating and better health. Most of us have begun well-intentioned New Years› resolution-type approaches that are unsustainable and quickly abandoned. Kari correctly proposes a very sustainable cycle of renewing relationships with food, support, and readiness. And I love how she ends on *Enjoy*! So many well-intentioned diets flounder because they are simply not enjoyable. I love how Kari invites us to enjoy the process, the small steps, and sharing with those around us.

Two thumbs-ups and Bravo!

Mark Nelson, MD

Acknowledgments

This book couldn't have been written without the encouragement of my family and friends. I'd like to thank Roger for his support and belief in me—the man I've shared a life with for over thirty years.

Thank you, Victoria Candland, for assisting me with your amazing editing skills and for giving me confidence. I'd also like to thank Briana Smith; Claine Snow, JD, PhD; Marilyn Faulkner; Megan McPhie; Robert G. Allen; Sherry Ledakis, JD; Mark Nelson, MD; and Susan Lane, MD, for your proofreading and for giving me your wisdom and advice while the book materialized.

I'm grateful for all those who came before me who wrote books, conducted research, created articles, and put their voices out there for me to learn from. Without your time and effort, I never would have been able to put together the facts and details contained in this book.

Lastly, I'd like to thank all the clients I have had the good pleasure of working with over the decades. *Eat Real Food and Love It: 6 Steps to Help You Crave Healthy Eating* was written with your struggles in mind.

Introduction

This book isn't another diet plan, another fad diet, or a way to lose *x* amount of weight in thirty days. *Eat Real Food and Love It* will help you understand the way you currently take care of your health and how you can use this awareness to move down the path of real, lasting, long-term wellness. *This book can help you find a way to overcome the desire for foods and beverages that have a negative impact on your health.*

Through my personal experience and throughout my career, I've learned that transforming eating and drinking habits is complicated. The process isn't easy. It can be messy and frustrating. But one thing is certain: changing what you desire to eat is possible. I did it, and I have seen the change in thousands of other people. Learning to crave healthy foods can help increase your quality of life, but it doesn't happen overnight. Be patient; the process takes time. Your brain has billions of neurons (nerve cells) that need to be reprogrammed and old memories that need to be overridden. For some people, the task can take several months; others may require a good two years or longer.

After working with many people over my career, I have identified a sequence of behaviors I have used and that have worked for my clients to turn them toward nature. Learning to eat and drink healthily can be achieved through a series of guiding steps that spell out the word *NATURE*. These steps build on each other and give you the power to change. Here are the six steps that can help you crave nature:

N
Notice the foods you are eating each day.

A
Analyze the contents of the foods you eat
before putting them in your body.

T
Train your brain to form new positive connections with nature's foods.

U
Unite clean eating with exercise and meditation
to form a healthy, natural lifestyle.

R
Renew your positive relationship with nature's foods
every day, even when you revert to old cravings.

E
Enjoy nature's foods as they become a permanent
part of your eating routine.

Eat Real Food and Love It contains action steps at the beginning and end of each chapter. These are designed to help you develop a symbiotic relationship with nature's foods. Keep this book close to you and reread it often throughout your process of change.

The result of following nature's steps is freedom. When you automatically crave healthy foods out of pleasure—not because you're on a diet—you're free from the ball and chain that hooks you into wanting foods and beverages that wear down your body and brain. Below are ten outcomes of following the nature steps:

NATURE Step Outcomes

1. No diet program is needed.
2. Your body is at a healthy weight.
3. You have mental clarity and energy.
4. Hunger is satisfied by the foods you choose.
5. You desire to eat foods that nourish you most of the time.
6. Your thoughts automatically choose nature's foods.
7. You feel fuller longer.
8. You enjoy endless combinations of amazing flavors.
9. You treat yourself in the highest regard through personalized nourishment, movement, and meditation.
10. You feel more connected to the Creator, who made nature's foods for you.

In *Eat Real Food and Love It*, we will discuss how foods from nature are designed to attract you to consume them but why you may be drawn to junk food instead. We will touch on the topic of epigenetics, which shows how genes interact and affect chemical changes in your cells. We will look at how your body slowly deteriorates from exposure to chemicals and at the history behind our current wheat industry. We will look at how your tongue can be manipulated to get you hooked on processed foods. We'll learn about brain chemistry and memory, and explore how industries create processed foods and beverages with the primary goal of enticing you to consume. We'll look at habit formation and transformation. We will explore an organized food guide, Nature's Food Selection Guide, which provides a way to eat that assists your desire to eat real foods. We'll touch on food addictions and how relationships are formed with food. We will review how nature's food can be enjoyable. And finally, we will provide you with a multistep process designed to help you *want* to consume nature's foods.

Eat Real Food and Love It is about helping you understand your taste preferences so you can decide whether you want to embrace them or change them. If you want to break away from habits, compulsions, and desires to eat foods or drink beverages that are negatively affecting your body, then this book is for you. Walk with me on a journey to change your palate and begin to desire foods and beverages produced by nature, which I will refer to in the book as "nature's foods" meaning "real foods." Lose the desire to consume foods and beverages that have been reconfigured, chemically manipulated, processed in a factory, run through conveyor belts, and pumped or dropped into strategically labeled packages, which I will refer to in the book as "synthetic foods."

There's nothing like necessity to get you to crave nature's foods from the earth and help you restore your health and weight. So, what do you want or need? Maybe you want to be slimmer, or maybe you're more concerned about specific health problems like diabetes or high blood pressure. Maybe you want to be more energetic. Maybe you need to be a healthy role model for your children, coworkers, students, patients, family, or friends. Maybe you just want to feel better. Can you identify with any of these needs or desires? If so, let's get started on your journey toward nature and a love for real food.

STEP 1

N
Notice the foods you are eating each day.

Chapter 1

Notice Your Current Patterns of Eating

The human body is a work of art, and so are foods grown in nature. When intertwined together, nature is at its finest.

Step 1: Notice

Gather Data

Your first step toward craving nature's foods is to notice and pay attention to what you are currently eating and drinking. When you do this, you start to recognize your recent state of eating. Only when you understand what your current patterns and habits are can you begin to make plans to change.

Elizabeth's Journey toward Eating Nature's Foods

Years ago a client (I'll call her "Elizabeth") came to me, wanting my professional advice about how to lose weight again. This was her fifth attempt. She had been successful at losing weight and keeping it off for several months while working with specialists, but she had always slipped back into eating behaviors that eventually caused her to regain the weight. She had tried multiple diets over the years, paying attention to whatever diet fad was popular at the time. Recently, Elizabeth had started seeing a trend toward plant-based eating, which she tried, but because of her active family and social life, she found herself not consuming as many plants as she thought she would.

After having Elizabeth record what she was eating through a food record, we discovered that Elizabeth mostly ate a lot of foods like bagels, fast-food sandwiches, pizza, burgers, tacos, chips, crackers, ribs, french fries, candy bars, cupcakes, and brownies. She drank coffee drinks, regular and diet sodas, wine, and beer. These foods and beverages were abundant at almost every event and gathering she attended, and although there were healthier foods available, she found herself indulging in the foods and beverages she was regularly exposed to.

Throughout the years of yo-yo weight cycling and counseling, Elizabeth concluded that the underpinnings of her poor food cravings weren't psychological. She didn't have emotional baggage she was trying to suppress with food. She couldn't identify with needing food to cope with life. She wasn't a victim of sexual abuse, which may have caused her to subconsciously want to put on a protective weight shell. She simply said to me, "The reason I'm overweight is that I *like* to eat and drink."

"Good!" I responded. "Then let's change the foods and beverages you like to eat and drink."

Elizabeth looked at me and said, "In all the years I've tried to lose weight and keep it off, no one has ever presented that concept."

Elizabeth needed to create new sensory habits and patterns to help her permanently crave healthy foods and beverages, and she was ready for the journey. She kept recording what she was eating and drinking, making small adjustments to her diet little by little. Over time Elizabeth changed from craving the highly processed foods she frequently ate, which were full of additives, fillers, and preservatives, to eating clean foods directly from nature. Eventually, her weight dropped from 186 pounds (84.5 kg) to 140 to 145 pounds (64 to 66 kg), and she has maintained that weight range now for more than four years. She has more energy, sleeps better, and can join friends on hiking trips she couldn't do at 186 pounds when she had constant knee pain. She is maximizing her body's function through food.

Throughout the book, we'll take a look at Elizabeth's progression toward nature. There are many stories similar to hers. Maybe you can relate.

Why Don't We Automatically Eat More Plants?

In your first step to wanting to eat real foods from nature, pay attention to what you are currently eating and drinking. You may discover that the number of foods you consume out of packages outnumber the ones you eat from nature. Although we were born into a world where delicious and healthful fruits, vegetables, nuts, seeds, legumes, and grains abound, these foods are easily bypassed because they are less convenient, sometimes more expensive, and at times less flavorful than processed foods, which set off fireworks in the brain. It's startling that despite the health attributes of edible plants, most people don't eat a lot of them. Studies show that almost 60 percent of calories in the US diet come from ultra-processed foods (which I call "synthetic" foods) that use additives and typically contain little or no intact real foods and are ready to eat, drink, or heat up.[2] That means over half of what Americans eat are foods pumped out by companies rather than by Mother Nature.

There are several reasons why people don't eat healthy foods, but many people choose food today due to its convenience, cost, and taste. If you take note of the last time you ate processed food instead something from nature, you may recognize that your choice was based on the fact that one was quicker, cheaper, and more exciting to your taste buds. Through experience, you probably remember the blissful flavor that came from a convenience food instead of a food picked in nature. Also, if you wonder whether people don't understand the difference between nature's foods and processed foods, just think. If you ask a child whether a carrot or a cheese puff is healthier, the child will likely point to the carrot. But what if I asked you the same question? Would you say the carrot? Hopefully you would. Now if you were offered each of them to eat, why would you choose a cheese puff if you *know* a carrot is healthier?

The answers to basic nutrition questions are obvious to people of all ages, suggesting that a lack of nutrition knowledge isn't the reason behind poor food choices. Like Elizabeth, processed foods hook you into consuming them because they can be acquired easily, are low priced, and taste amazing. Manufacturers know that when they combine great taste with low price and convenience, their products sell. Therefore, inherent appetites for natural foods are manipulated and overridden by affordable, highly automated, mutilated, tainted, reconfigured, and strategically crafted foods and beverages. As a result, when you eat foods equivalent to cheese puffs and skip nature's foods like carrots, you miss out on the opportunity to receive protective shields that can safeguard your health.

In this first step, simply notice your food choices. When you do this, you start to recognize and understand what your patterns are, and you can begin to make plans to change if you need to.

In Chapter 2, we'll look at nature's foods and what they have to offer.

Chapter 2

Notice What Nature's Foods Do for You

To operate a computer, you need to move your mouse around to access the different icons and features of your operating system. It's the navigation that commands and instructs the computer to work the way you want it to. Food works in the same way. It provides the ingredients and instructions your body needs so it can know how to run. For example, if you eat food from nature like a handful of carrots, the fiber (a main constituent) lands in your stomach, filling it up and causing it to distend, which instructs your brain and body to stop eating.

Nature's foods allow your body and mind to function at full capacity by defending and protecting your cells instead of attacking them. They also keep your body at an appropriate weight for your frame, assist you in healing from disease, and allow you to have the energy your body needs not only to operate but also to flourish throughout your life span.

List 2A shows a sampling of foods I consider to be nature's foods. An organized guide showing how to work these foods into your lifestyle is found in Chapter 25. (Note that every time "nature's food" is mentioned throughout the book, it refers to "real" or "clean" food and includes beverages.)

Nature's Foods

- Organically grown fruits and vegetables
- Unsweetened, sprouted, organic whole grains and legumes
- Unsweetened organic milk alternatives
- Cold-pressed oils
- Unsweetened nuts and seeds

Occasional Animal Products (Once or Twice per Week, if Desired)

- Lean, free-range, grass-fed animal or plant proteins
- Wild-caught fish
- Hormone-free, unsweetened, organic milk or yogurt

See specific food ideas in Chapter 25.

Disclaimer: Whole food, plant-based eating with minimal animal products is the preferred way to eat. The animal products listed above are the highest grade, but ideally, it's recommended that you consume them sparingly or not at all.

If you think your budget doesn't allow for many of the items above, consider that when your money goes toward nature's foods, you'll reduce your purchases of synthetic foods, which will help your budget. Your body will also be healthier, which means you will ultimately spend less money on doctor's visits and experience fewer health complications caused by unhealthy eating.

Nature's Food: Why We Need It

On the day you were born, you began seeking food. That's because your brain's number one job is to make sure you stay alive, and your brain knows food is needed for survival. Yet as noted earlier, statistics show that 60 percent (or more) of the foods consumed are ultra-processed, not foods from nature. To sway the pendulum closer to nature's side, understanding the quantity and quality of food you eat is essential. Let's review the purpose of plants and see whether you're benefiting from their healing properties.

Plants are designed to heal, repair, and sustain your body. They deliver powerful nutrients and bioactive compounds with every bite. As a first step to craving healthy foods, notice what you're eating and note whether your food choices are in a harmonious state with nature. Are you taking advantage of the goodness grown outdoors for your nourishment?

For thousands of years, humans have lived off the land, consuming exclusively what nature produced. For thousands of years, plants have nourished and kept the human body strong. Now we understand that our bodies have a symbiotic relationship with plants. From breathing to eating, your body needs plants—and they need you. Every time you exhale, you put carbon dioxide into the air. Plants nearby, as if their leaves were lungs, breathe it in, and in return they create oxygen for *you* to breathe. This same interdependency is seen when you eat plants. During digestion and absorption, plants assist in the health and function of your body, and *they* mutually benefit when you eat them. Let's explore this concept further.

Nature's Foods: Why They Need *You* to Eat Them

To better understand how plants benefit from our eating them, let's take a look at their life cycle and the chemical processes they go through when they ripen. If you have ever bitten into a fruit or vegetable that was too green or not ripe enough, your mouth probably told you the unripe produce was unpalatable. Maybe you spat it back out. Plants need time to ripen before they can help you. Plants you end up consuming like apples, peaches, peppers, mangos, and avocados give off signals that they are ready to be eaten after they mature. Similar to the internal changes humans experience during puberty, wherein the pituitary gland secretes luteinizing hormone (LH), which activates the secretion of estrogen and testosterone, plants secrete hormones unique to them like auxin, cytokinin, gibberellin, ethylene (a gaseous hormone), and abscisic acid. [160] These hormones are released during the plant version of puberty and work not only to influence the plant's growth but also to transform it from inedible to edible.

At the onset of plant puberty when plant hormones are secreted, they internally burst and create a big-bang activation of growth enzymes. Assisting the process are the plants' phytonutrients (the prefix *phyto* is of Greek origin and means "plant"). The phytonutrients are the plants' protective shields they use to protect themselves from invaders, ultraviolet radiation, harsh weather, predators, insects, pollution, toxins and altered colors, smells, and flavors. Like humans, they have to defend themselves from threats to their survival.

When there is a cascade of new puberty enzymes on board, plants undergo a variety of changes. One of the activated enzymes plants secrete is amylase, which internally breaks down starch into sugar to sweeten the plants. Other enzymes knock down the plants' pectin, encouraging them to soften and release a fragrant, appealing smell. [85] During the ripening process, the activation of enzymes causes the pigments of chlorophyll to break down, [56] removing the camouflaged green color. After puberty, the plant's adult version is primed and ready to transfer their phytonutrients to your body when you eat them.

To illustrate plant maturity further, let's take a look at the ripening process of a tomato. A tomato that starts off green on the vine will during "puberty" receive signals from its hormones that it is time to ripen. The signals will cause the tomato to turn from its original green color—the color that enables the tomato to disguise itself into its surroundings—to a beautiful red color that beckons the eye. The tomato will also appeal to your sense of smell by emitting a sweet tomato fragrance when it is ripe and ready to be eaten. Essentially, at that point in the ripening process, the tomato is saying, "Come and get me" (in an anthropomorphic manner of speaking, of course).

The reason why tomatoes (and all edible plants) want to appeal to your senses, especially sight, is because they *want* to attract your hungry eye. Like humans, plants need to multiply to ensure their survival. They can perpetuate their species only if they spread their seeds far and wide. This happens when plants are consumed by mobile beings (an animal or you!), and their seeds run through the body of the host and out the other end. Plants nourish your body in exchange for their seed being carried and deposited remotely. Through excrement, plant seeds are deposited throughout the land. That's why once a plant matures and ripens, it gives off signals that it is ready to be consumed. Plants need to preserve their genus. Humans and plants need each other for survival.

Fiber Cleanse

Of all the gifts plants give your human body, one of the greatest is fiber. Your body uses the plant fibers found in the cell walls, peels, and the seeds of the vegetables, fruits, nuts, seeds, legumes, and grains to scrub out the waste materials that build up in your intestines. Think of fiber as a brush that scours your intestinal tract and moves waste material through your twenty feet (six meters) of small intestines and five feet (1.5 meters) of large intestines and out. [82] Fiber contains a health-promoting aspect of nature's foods that is essential for the proper functioning of your digestive tract.

In this first step, notice, I encourage you to gather data on what foods you're eating. As part of the process, also keep track of how much fiber you consume. A range of 25-38 grams of fiber a day is sure to keep your intestinal tract cleansed. Besides fiber, plants have a lot more to offer. The reach of plants from your digestive tract affects every cell in your body down to the smallest units in your body, your atoms.

Your Body Makeup

One of my favorite classes in college was biochemistry. I was fascinated with all the components and processes that made up the human body. What I learned is that the body is made up of matter and energy, and the hierarchy begins with the atom. When two or more atoms are linked together by a bond, they are called "molecules." Molecules are bound together by electrons, which can attract or repulse other molecules. Your body is a system of molecules packed tightly due to these attractions and repulsions. This package makes up your body's cells, which are specialized chemical factories. Your cells group together to form tissues that shape your organs, which make up your organ systems and ultimately design you as an entire human being.

Diagram A
illustrates the progression of your body from an atom.

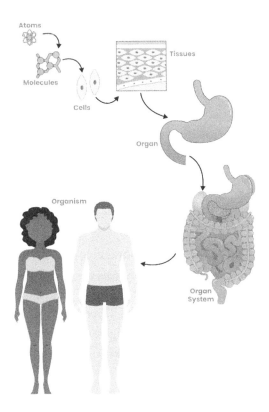

Your body is constantly breaking down and building up molecules, a process called your "metabolism." In every moment of your life, proteins are building, and cells are dividing. Deep inside each of your body's cells, these functions are ongoing, even as you read this book. Your human body is so vast and complex that if you unraveled all the deoxyribonucleic acid (DNA) packed tightly in your cells, it's estimated that, if laid end to end, it would span about two times the diameter of the solar system, which is 7 billion miles (11,265,408,000 km) long. [154]

If you study the complexity of how your DNA, enzymes, genes, and other structures function within your trillions of body cells, you will see that you have an extremely busy world of operations going on, orchestrated by a sophisticated and complex genetic coding system. [2] It's a fascinating internal microscopic world of assembly that makes you unchangeable and unique. Because your body is so complicated, all the intertwined mechanisms involved in running your system are beyond our complete understanding at this point. However, from the slow growth of your toenails to the rapid fire of the neurons in your brain, all your bodily functions need the correct amount and type of fuel source. This is where nutrition comes in. *What you bring into your body matters. Everything you take in contains ingredients that either contribute to the intricate systems that run your body or degrade them.* Since you were born into this world to eat what the earth provides, edible plants were simultaneously designed with the correct ingredients to run your body.

Antioxidants: How Nature's Foods Assist Your Cells

With similar complexity to the human body, nature's foods are first composed of atoms that contain electrons. Diagram B shows how both human beings and plants are formed from atoms.

Diagram B

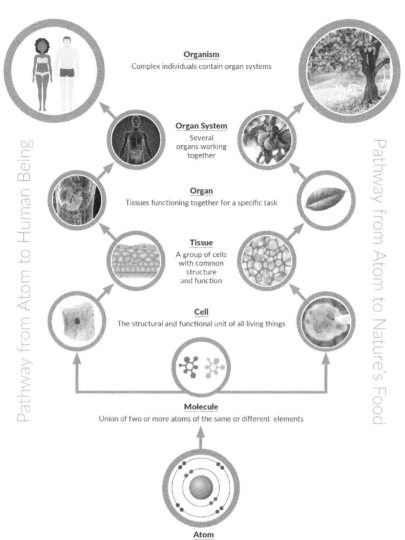

When you consume plants, they contribute to your life force by donating repair electrons in a process called "antioxidation." Most of my clients are aware of antioxidants but don't really know how they work. Here is an explanation I hope will make the process more understandable.

Antioxidation occurs in the electrons that orbit the atoms inside your body cells. Each atom in your body stays stable in its location by electrons that surround or orbit the atoms, and these electrons travel in pairs. Diagram C illustrates how electrons orbiting the atom are arranged in pairs.

Diagram C

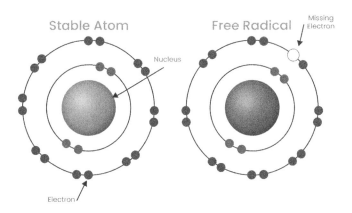

In Diagram C, the "stable atom" has a pair of electrons in its first orbit and eight electrons in its outer orbit, but the "free radical" atom has lost an electron. It's this roaming electron that is called a "free radical." It travels around, looking for another companion. A free radical will attack molecules and try to steal electrons from them so it can pair up again. The stealing of an electron is called "oxidative stress" (or "oxidation"), and once the stealing begins, a cascade of robbery can ignite throughout your atoms and impair the function of the molecule. [120]

Damage is seen over time when an overabundance of free radicals is formed and there is a shortage of antioxidants. Free radicals can form from processed foods, especially processed meats like bacon, sausage, and salami. They are also produced from pesticides, air pollution, cigarette smoke, alcohol, high blood sugar levels, sun exposure radiation, and/or antioxidant deficiencies—caused by not bringing in enough of nature's foods. Aging also increases your exposure to free-radical producers. Their damaging effects can be seen on your skin as wrinkles and/or in your body in the form of diseases like cancer, inflammatory joint disease, atherosclerosis, asthma, diabetes, senile dementia, and degenerative eye disease. These exposures cause your electrons to become unpaired, detach from their partners, and run amok, producing more free-radical damage.

Fighting off free-radical damage is where phytonutrients and antioxidants come in. When you consume foods grown on trees, vines, bushes, and roots, you consume plants that have developed defensive strategies. Your body in turn receives these nutritious shields of protection, which are electrons that stabilize and reduce oxidative stress in your cells. If you don't bring in nature's foods, your cells won't receive stabilizing electrons and will have a significantly weakened ability for repair when free-radical damage occurs.

Diagram D shows an electron from a plant being donated to restabilize the cell.

Diagram D

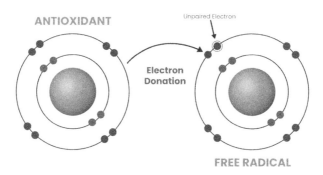

Antioxidants from plants function by donating electrons. By stabilizing the order of electrons, antioxidants prevent the damage that might otherwise cascade throughout your cells, causing mutations. After you consume plants, they happily give you electrons to replace any that are missing in your cells. This puts an end to the electron-stealing reaction and keeps your cells functioning healthfully.

Table 1 lists a few well-studied phytonutrients with powerful health benefits that contribute electrons for antioxidation.

Table 1

Phytonutrient	Color(s)	Found in These Foods	Benefit
Carotenoids: Alpha-carotene, beta-carotene, lycopene	Bright red, red, pink, orange, and yellow	Carrots, sweet potatoes, dark-green leafy vegetables, tomatoes	Alpha and beta-carotenes: Convert to vitamin A, which helps your immune system work properly. Lycopene has been linked to a lower risk of prostate cancer. All carotenoids are high in antioxidants that protect eyes from disease by absorbing damaging blue light that enters the eye. [7,6]
Flavonoids: Catechins, flavonols, quercetin	Multi-colored	Almost all fruits and vegetables, particularly apples, citrus fruits, berries, tomatoes, romaine lettuce, green tea, 72 percent or more of dark chocolate, and legumes	High in antioxidants designed to absorb molecules to prevent them from becoming reactive. They act as an antihistamine and have antimicrobial, memory, and mood-enhancing properties. [8]

Indoles	Green	Arugula, broccoli, brussels sprouts, cabbage, cauliflower, collard greens, and kale	They protect cells against cancer, particularly breast, cervical, and colorectal. They aid in fibromyalgia, have antiviral properties, detoxify intestines and liver, and balance hormone levels. [62]
Isothiocyanates: Glucoraphanin, Sulfora, and phane	Green, red, and white	Cruciferous vegetables like bok choy, cabbage, cauliflower, broccoli, brussels sprouts, kale, kohlrabi, turnips, radishes, rutabaga, and watercress	They protect cells against cancer, particularly cancers of the gastrointestinal and respiratory tracts. [109]
Lignans	Brown and orange	Seeds (flax, pumpkin, sunflower, poppy, sesame), whole grains, beans, and fruits (particularly berries)	They protect against estrogen-related cancers, particularly breast, prostate, and colon cancers. They support cardiovascular health and alleviate estrogen-dependent conditions such as osteoporosis and symptoms of menopause. [20]
Organosulfides	Green and white	Garlic, onions, and leeks	They protect against plaque buildup in the arteries and can prevent complications of diabetes and cardiovascular disease. [116]

Phytosterols	Brown	Seeds (sesame seed, sunflower seed), nuts (pistachios, pine nuts, almonds), wheat germ, bran (rice bran, corn bran, wheat bran), flour (soy flour, buckwheat flour, rye flour, whole-wheat flour), and soybeans	They compete for the same enzymes as cholesterol, preventing cholesterol from being absorbed. [162]

The phytonutrients from the plants listed in Table 1 have been scientifically found to enhance your immune system, provide antioxidants, ward off cancer, protect your eyes, stimulate the function of your brain by helping your moods and memory, protect your bones, fight against plaque buildup in your arteries, and help to normalize your cholesterol. These are all conditions you most likely ask a doctor to prevent or treat. Just think, by consuming more plants, you can save time and medical costs.

As we've established, plants can protect you by donating electrons from their living cells once you eat them. They are beckoning you to consume them so they can safeguard your body's cells and defend you against oxidation from free-radical damage. Gather data on how many plants you are eating and ask yourself with every bite or sip, "Is what I'm consuming contributing to the protection of my body cells?" If the answer is no, turn to nature's foods. Over time the hope is that you will begin saying yes more than no once your palate starts adjusting more toward the foods grown in nature.

Sledgehammers

When invaders come into your body in the form of processed foods, pesticides, air pollution, cigarette smoke or alcohol, it's as if there's a sledgehammer on the loose inside your cells. These invaders can cause oxidative damage and form free radicals. Free radicals can break apart valuable structures in your cells like proteins, cell membranes and your DNA. [117]

Diagram E

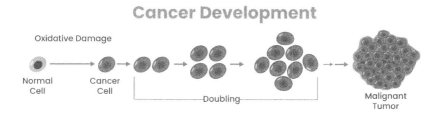

In Diagram E, the normal cell is damaged by free radicals running amok and causing oxidative damage. This can occur from a single contact to, or an accumulating effect of, the additives in synthetic foods. Oxidative damage in the normal cell affects the cell's DNA, [117] which causes a genetic change and a cancer cell. [88] If cancerous cells divide, they develop into tumors. If tumors find a blood supply, they start traveling around your body and forming cancerous communities. The wrecked cells take over the once-healthy cells, and tissues begin to die. Antioxidants from plant foods can halt the process of tumor formation by keeping your cells normal and healthy. They also boost your immune system and stop free radicals from causing damage to your cells. With antioxidants on board, you can stop cancer cells from proliferating. Real foods from nature are full of antioxidants designed to defend and protect your brain and body, not damage your DNA.

As previously noted, free radicals can act as sledgehammers inside your body cells. Therefore, consider the next time you put something equivalent to a cheese puff to your lips. Your trillions of body cells [137] are missing out on the opportunity to receive protective electron antioxidants, whereas when you eat carrots or other plant foods, you bring in electrons to protect your cells. Just like a house can handle only so many hits with a sledgehammer before it crashes, your body can withstand only a certain number of contaminants before it suffers. Over time free radicals produced by oxidative stress (like sledgehammers) break down the walls of your human cells and cause your body to spend energy detoxifying the unnatural additives that come into the body.

You can help stop the damage by bringing in antioxidant defenders. In the next chapter, we'll explore foods that have no stabilizing electrons on board—synthetic foods. We'll take a look at foods that have been handled, pulverized, and mixed with ample amounts of additives, preservatives, fat, sugar, and salt; these are foods that promote the sledgehammer effect.

Chapter 3

Notice the Ingredients in Synthetic Foods

Synthetic Foods

When nature's plant and animal foods are processed so they can be preserved and stocked on a store shelf, they become a huge source of revenue for manufacturers. My term for processed food, ultra-processed food, or junk food created by a chemical synthesis is "synthetic food." (Note that every time synthetic food is mentioned in this book, it includes beverages.)

> **Synthetic Foods**
>
> Packaged and bottled foods and beverages that are commercially prepared for ease of consumption can sit on a shelf for an extended period beyond their natural expiration period. These foods can include, but are not limited to, chips, cookies, crackers, pastries, doughnuts, processed meats, bacon, sausage, sauces, cereals, candy, creamers, convenience foods like microwavable meals, fast foods, white-flour products, packaged bars, sodas, alcoholic beverages, juices and sweetened drinks.

Most synthetic foods are calorie dense, which means they are high in calories but have low nutritional value. They have become the main staple of the standard American diet (SAD). The standard American diet (SAD) is in Wikipedia as a descriptor that defines a pattern of eating that includes high amounts of butter, corn, high-fructose corn syrup, dairy products, fried foods, high-sugar drinks, potatoes, prepackaged foods, and processed and red meats. [164] These foods are part of my synthetic food list.

Most people give up the amount of nature's foods they consume once their brains discover synthetic foods because they are affordable and taste too good to pass up. What may not be immediately apparent to them is that with a higher consumption of synthetic foods, they can quickly get hooked on them. Research continues to unfold that frequent and large quantities of calories from synthetic foods contribute to the compulsion to eat more and more of them—like drugs. That's because the same brain processes affected by drugs also control your eating and are involved with your thoughts, reward systems, and emotions. [115] And for survival purposes, because you're living in a day and age where you can acquire large quantities of easily accessible synthetic foods and beverages, your brain tells you to find them and consume them again and again. Therefore, if you want to take these foods out of your life, you need new skills to manage them. Following the NATURE steps in this book assists you on your journey away from craving foods that negatively affect your body and toward desiring more real foods.

Synthetic Ingredients

Food and beverage companies have worked for decades to refine their products in the hopes that your brain will continue to forage for the flavor of a particular food once you have tasted it. They work with a multibillion-dollar flavoring industry that strategically designs synthetic foods, hoping they will appeal to your brain. (More on the flavoring industry in Chapter 9.) Processed food and beverages today most often include only a small amount of ingredients sourced from nature, along with unhealthy ingredients.

Additionally, any ingredients that originate from nature in food products are often mutilated and mixed with additives and chemicals to increase their shelf life. When this happens, the nutritional value of the natural ingredient plummets, and the food's ability to anti-oxidize and protect your cells diminishes. Take, for example, the transformation of an ear of corn into the snack product I referred to earlier, cheese puffs. If you look at the ingredients listed on a bag of cheese puffs, these are the words you will find: "enriched corn meal (corn meal, ferrous sulfate, niacin, thiamin mononitrate, riboflavin, and folic acid), vegetable oil (corn, canola, and/or sunflower oil), cheese seasoning (whey, cheddar cheese [milk, cheese cultures, salt, enzymes], canola oil, maltodextrin [made from corn], salt, whey protein concentrate, monosodium glutamate, natural and artificial flavors, lactic acid, citric acid, artificial color [Yellow 6]), and salt."

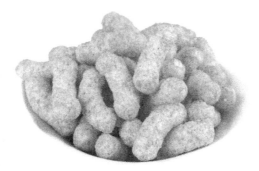

To make cheese puffs, the ear of the corn is shaved down, and the dried individual kernels are ground up and made into cornmeal. Then the cornmeal is combined with oil, cheese-flavored powder, and some water to create a paste-like dough. The dough is cooked and pressure-pushed through a mold to create an inflated, finger-shaped "puff." The puffs go through either a baking or frying process, in which they are sprayed with additional flavorings and seasonings and glistened with a bright-orange food coloring to make you believe they have cheese in them. They are then moved along a conveyor belt, where they are dropped into moisture-resistant plastic bags, which are heat-sealed into boxes and shipped to stores. [65]

By the time you put a cheese puff in your mouth, any nutrients your body would have received from the corn, the only redeeming food source, is gone. In fact, the puffs are full of ingredients that don't assist your body's defense systems and can cause your liver to do extra work filtering out unneeded food additives. Similar processing styles are involved with creating other synthetic foods like chips, cookies, crackers, pastries, doughnuts, processed meats, fries, sugary cereals, candy, lollipops, creamers, fast foods, white floured products, and packaged bars, to name a few. As you keep track of what you're eating, pay attention to the number of processed foods and beverages you consume. Do they outnumber the amount of nature's foods you eat?

Processing doesn't just occur in food products. Some beverages are nothing more than a blend of liquid chemicals. For example, here are the ingredients in a popular soft drink (soda): "sugar, concentrated orange juice, citric acid, natural flavors, sodium benzoate, caffeine (54 mg per 12 US fluid ounces or 350 ml), sodium citrate, erythorbic acid, gum arabic, calcium disodium EDTA, bromated vegetable oil, Yellow 5." Other than concentrated orange juice, this soda (along with other beverages like sport drinks and energy drinks) is an absolute nutrient wasteland. If the ingredients alone don't deter you from choosing something else, consider that in a twenty-ounce (0.6 liter) bottle, there are 290 calories and 77 grams of sugar. To make sense of the amount of sugar this is, consider the fact that there are four grams of sugar in every teaspoon. Seventy-seven divided by four equals 19.25. Therefore, one twenty-ounce bottle of this beverage has 19.25 teaspoons of sugar in it! Since sugar is the first and main ingredient in this soda, you are getting a large dose of it melted down and mixed with an entourage of chemicals with every sip. It's the same amount as if you went to a restaurant, ordered a large glass of water or mug of tea, and then dumped nineteen packets of sugar in it before you drank it.

Synthetic Ingredients

Synthetic ingredients sold on the global market are widely used in what we consume today. A few popular flavor enhancers and their associated risk are listed in Table 2. See if you notice any of these ingredients in the foods you eat.

Table 2

Additive	Food Products (Read the ingredients on the label to verify whether the additive is present.)	Risk
Sugar and high-fructose corn syrup	• Cereals • Condiments • Crackers • Jams and jellies • Juices • Kids' foods • Salad dressings • Soft drinks • Yogurts	Overconsumption of added sugars (sucrose or table sugar and high-fructose corn syrup) has been associated with an increased risk of fatty liver disease, [74] heart disease, and death from cardiovascular causes. [39] Sugar has also been linked to an increased risk of breast cancer, [75] tooth and gum disease, and obesity. [36]
MSG (monosodium glutamate)	Foods containing MSG: • Bone broths • Corn starch • Corn syrup • Cured meats (ham, sausage) • Fish sauce • Low-fat products • Malted barley (breads, beer) • Matured cheeses (Parmesan, Roquefort) • Soy sauce and soy protein • Vitamin-enriched products Ingredients containing MSG" • Bouillon, broth, stock • Brewer's yeast • Natural flavor • Maltodextrin	MSG or food additive number E620 has possible toxic effects including central nervous system disorder, obesity, disruptions in adipose (fat) tissue physiology, reproductive malfunctions, and kidney damage. [110]

Sodium benzoates	· Fruit juices · Jams · Juice drinks · Pickles · Marinades · Salad dressings · Sauces · Soft drinks	Evidence suggests that a high intake of sodium benzoate may be linked to attention deficit-hyperactivity disorder (ADHD) in children. Short-term consumption of sodium benzoate can impair memory performance and increase brain oxidative stress in mice. Sodium benzoate is a widely used preservative and antimicrobial substance in many foods and soft drinks. [81]
Acesulfame potassium (Ace-K)	• Baked goods • Candies • Frozen desserts • Juice drinks • Soft drinks	Acesulfame potassium (Ace-K) is one of the most commonly used artificial sweeteners for foods and beverages. Mice fed a low carbohydrate diet with Ace-K for four weeks showed an increase in water intake and a decrease in short-term and object cognitive memory. [66]
Federal Food, Drug & Cosmetic Act (FD&C) color dyes such as blue, green, red, orange, and yellow	• Baked goods • Breakfast bars • Candy • Cereal • Chocolate • Frozen desserts • Icing • Instant pudding • Ketchup • Marshmallows • Mustard	The amount of artificial food colors (AFCs) consumed, according to the Food and Drug Administration, increased more than five-fold from 1950 (12 mg/capita/day) to (68 mg/capita/day). Since 1950 there have been studies of adverse behavioral reactions such as hyperactivity in children. Studies that used 50 mg or more of AFCs showed a

	• Pickles • Salad dressing • Soft drinks	greater negative effect on more children than those who used less. Three dyes—Red 40, Yellow 5, and Yellow 6—account for 90 percent of all dyes used. [145]
Sulfites	• Beer • Canned goods • Dried fruit • Juices • Meats • Processed fish • Seafood • Wine	Consumption of sulfites have been shown to damage beneficial bacteria in the gut microbiome. [70] Diseases related to damaged beneficial bacteria include chronic inflammation and obesity. [136]
Nitrates, nitrites	• Bacon • Canned meat • Corned beef • Ham • Hot dogs • Jerky • Salami • Sandwich meats • Sausages	Nitrate and nitrite compounds are believed to play a role in the development of colorectal cancer (CRC). The cooking of nitrite-containing meat is one of the major sources of carcinogens. [22] [170]

Since there are more than 12,000 additives and synthetic ingredients in our consumable products, [125] the ones shown in the table are a small sample of what's being put in our foods and beverages. These additives have slowly crept into the food supply over the years to improve texture, consistency, preservation, and flavor. Bear in mind that all these additives are intended to increase the sale of the product, not increase your health. Your best defense is to develop a palate for nature's foods so you will choose to avoid ingesting unwanted additives. In the next chapter, we'll look at how nature's foods can positively affect your DNA *and* the DNA of your offspring.

Chapter 4

Notice the Findings from Epigenetics and Nutrigenomics

In the United States, ultra-processed foods are available 24-7. This combination of great taste, low price, and convenience allows for ongoing indulgence. Let's take a deeper look into why we should be careful.

Epigenetics: Mice Are What Their Mothers Ate

Scientists are learning more and more that on a cellular level, processed foods are not only contributing to chronic diseases like diabetes and obesity but also affecting your gene expression, altering your DNA, and quite possibly changing the DNA you pass on to your children. There is an emerging field of study called "epigenetics," which is a branch of biology that studies how genes interact and can affect chemical changes in your cells. (*Epi* means "over or above," and "genetics" involves your genes and heredity.) Like an on or off switch, some of your genes are turned on or active, and some are off or inactive. The active genes are the ones your body uses for functioning. Epigeneticists are learning that foods affect how your cells read your genes to make appropriate proteins for your body. They are also discovering that when positive nutritional modifications are made, various genetic mutations can be reversed.

One of the first epigenetic experiments to shed light on how powerful food choices can be was an experiment that showed how a mother's diet during pregnancy affected the gene expression of her offspring. [104] In the experiment, it was discovered that when an unhealthy, overweight mother mouse consumed the supplements folic acid (the manufactured form of vitamin B_9 or folate) and choline, it ignited a gene that prompted her offspring to switch from the prevalence of being obese to being thin and healthy. This was accomplished by activating a genetic pathway called "methylation." Methyl groups that trigger methylation are found in nature's foods and are absent in synthetic foods. During pregnancy, after the overweight mouse's methyl pathways were turned on from the folic acid and choline supplements, the mouse passed the effects down to her offspring. When the pups were born, the methyl groups shut off an agouti gene, which would have made her pups prone to obesity, cancer, and diabetes. [140] Diagram F shows the lifelong effect the mother's folic acid and choline intake had on her pups.

Diagram F

On/Off

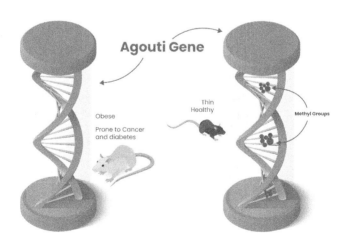

It's amazing to see the power of methylation. By receiving their mom's methyl groups, the pups' body chemistry changed from obese and prone to cancer and diabetes to thin and healthy for a life span. These results show the power of nutrition and that the diet of a pregnant mouse can influence the health of her offspring.

Although experiments on mice don't directly translate to humans, the same methylation that happened in the pregnant mouse applies in our nutrition. Clearly you can't control what was consumed while you were in your mother's womb, but you can bring in methyl groups now. You can make the switch anytime and widely bring in an abundance of methyl groups from nature's foods throughout your life span to help assist the function of your cells. For example, instead of taking the choline and folate supplements given to the pregnant, overweight mouse, eat good sources of choline, folate, and a multitude of other nutrients every day from nature's foods. Folate is found in leafy, green vegetables, sunflower seeds, citrus fruits, and beans. Choline is found in soybeans, mushrooms, kidney beans, quinoa, brussels sprouts, and broccoli. The next time you eat a green, leafy salad, throw in some orange wedges, mushrooms, kidney beans, soy beans, and/or sunflower seeds. You will enjoy a dose of methyl groups that are defending your DNA. And if you happen to be pregnant while eating this salad, you could be saving your descendants from a lifetime of potential obesity or disease.

If obesity genes can be turned off in mice, epigeneticists may one day uncover how to inactivate obesity and other problematic genes in humans. Although epigeneticists aren't quite there yet, the solution—to consume nature's foods—is simple. You can train your palate to desire foods that contain phytonutrients and methyl groups and give your cells the opportunity to combat obesity and disease. Keep walking with me on a journey to adjust your palate and create a desire for nature's foods.

Nutrigenomics: The Way

Another scientific field that applies to nutrition, still in its infancy, is called "nutrigenomics." [103] In the field of nutrigenomics, scientists study how foods affect our gene expression. There is a revolution in the nutrition field, and experts are striving to better understand the interactions between genes and nutrition and how they impact the health of each person uniquely. You may one day be able to understand how each food, beverage, additive, preservative, or chemical will affect each of your individual body cells and develop a personalized nutrition plan. By knowing your genotype or a portion of your genetic makeup, professionals in the field are looking to deliver an optimal nutrition plan specifically tailored to you. You may be able to discern how each substance you consume impacts the expression of your genes for good or bad.

Scientists in the nutrigenomics field have been sorting through a vast amount of data, developing experiments, and working on data storage to more fully understand how molecules in the human body interact with nutrients. [105] Perhaps advancements aren't further along in this field because, as with any business, there needs to be funding. Clinical nutrition research projects are typically funded through grants from financial backers with an invested interest in food and health. There is an ongoing need for sponsors.

As we make our shift to nature's food and our wallets show that change, the field of nutrigenomics will continue to emerge, and we're sure to see personalized nutrition plans custom-made to each person. I'm excited to see that day.

Chapter 5

Notice Summary, Recommendations, and Action Steps

My "Notice" Experience: Your Needs Are Unique

Looking back to how I progressed from consuming large amounts of synthetic foods to desiring nature's foods (most of the time), I began paying attention to how many fruits and vegetables I was consuming in a twenty-four-hour period. I realized that once I learned about phytonutrients and antioxidants and had a better understanding of their importance, I felt drawn to improve my diet. I knew that my cells needed fruits and vegetables, and even though I initially didn't have a palate for them, my internal wisdom encouraged me to nourish my cells. For me it was much easier to like and want to eat nature's food once I was educated about their benefits.

Here's one trick I used to notice my food and get to the point where I wanted to improve my health; every time I ate real food from nature, like a roasted vegetable, I put some awareness and focus on it. I consciously observed the mixture of its colors and imagined the abundance of phytonutrients and antioxidants in it. I closed my eyes and conceptualized how the vegetables I was eating were donating their protective armor and methyl groups to my trillions of body cells. I could see them internally defending and protecting my cells. My reward for eating the vegetables was feeling leaner, more energetic, and altogether healthier. By eating the vegetables, I perceived that I was nourishing myself at the healthiest level possible while creating an army of defenders as a wall of protection around my intestinal tract. As my health started changing for the better, it was easier to keep going. I noticed that I was having fewer mood swings because I was nurturing my body with foods that kept my blood sugar stable. I started feeling more vibrant and less lethargic. I sailed through my workouts, and my clothes fit me well. I stopped having to flip-flop from my fat clothes to my skinny ones. Throughout the process of observing my eating, I started believing more in healthy foods. I had the impression that the foods were creating a healthy impact, and my suspicion helped me to continue down the path of making better food choices.

My transition to nature's foods at first was difficult. It wasn't an epiphany or one-time event; rather, it was a process of experiences. Through trial and error, I brought produce into my world. Even to this day, I have to consciously organize my time to cut up a cucumber or carrot and grab an avocado or a "to-go" pack of guacamole rather than rely on my prior go-to chocolate bar. Eating from nature takes more time, effort, and planning, but nowadays I put the effort into it because of the health and energy I receive when I do so. Moreover, once I started to reap the benefits of healthful eating—like better skin, more energy, and fewer illnesses—it was easier to continue. *The healthier I ate, the more I wanted to eat healthily.*

Highlights to "Notice": The First Step to Reclaiming Natural Eating

- You have a symbiotic relationship with nature's food. You need it, and it needs you.
- Synthetic foods are artificially developed to entice you to eat *them*. (There's more on this topic in the next section, "Analyze.")
- The free radicals from synthetic foods and beverages act like sledgehammers. In your body, free radicals can cause a breakdown of structures inside your cells, leading to disease.
- Nature's foods and beverages can restore oxidative damage by donating electrons to repair free radical damage and stop a chain reaction of electron stealing. This protects your body's cells.

Notice Recommendations and Action Steps

Nature's foods are full of the nutrients that protect your body cells. However, as demonstrated previously, once nature's foods and beverages are processed, their original healing properties are stripped, and they no longer offer protection. When corn is made into cheese puffs or oranges are first made into concentrated orange juice and then into soda, all the goodness in them is essentially gone. Bite per bite, begin to notice the health-sustaining effect of real food. Conversely, recognize there is an unfortunate sledgehammer-like impact of synthetic foods.

Step 1: Gather Data

In this first chapter - "Notice"—your first step in desiring nature's foods is to notice what you are eating. Pay attention to what foods you are choosing. In my experience people who keep some kind of record double their weight loss and are able to make better changes in their health because they're aware of the eating and drinking practices that need to be adjusted.

If you think this sounds obvious, what I have realized from working with thousands of clients over the years is that once you establish your likes and dislikes, your eating and drinking become automatic habits. When I ask them, "Name everything you ate and drank yesterday," the vast majority of people can't even remember with exactness all they consumed the day before. That's because their brains were preoccupied during eating and busy with other activities. What was being eaten wasn't registered as an eating event.

The best way to notice what you are eating and drinking is to write down what you consume or at minimum, mentally keep track of everything you eat. If there is a cookie on the counter and you throw it in your mouth, write it down. You can also enter the information in one of the many devices like a Fitbit or Apple Watch or use an online tracking program or app on your phone like MyFitnessPal, MyPlate, or SparkPeople. Recording your foods puts awareness and focus on your current state of eating.

Record what's going in your mouth five days a week. When you get a good handle on it, drop down to three days a week. If that seems like too much ongoing, even once a week can help. The clients of mine who record their food intake make the fastest change from consuming synthetic foods to eating and drinking natural foods. Their brains become aware of previously programmed habitual patterns, which allow them to shift their focus on new strategies to break from repetitive acts. Notice the transitions going on within you as you progress on your road to change.

During your food and beverage tracking, remember to keep track of how many plant foods and the amount of fiber you eat. Shoot for twenty-five to fifty grams of fiber per day. During this process, be specific.

Here is an example of a food journal, showing where Elizabeth (mentioned in Chapter 1) started and where her progression is now:

Elizabeth's Food and Beverage Journal

	Beginning in October	Transitional April	Nature's Eating October
Breakfast	• Café mocha, 12 oz. • Plain bagel, 3.8 oz. • Cream cheese, 2 Tbsp, (Starbucks)	• Coffee with cream, 8 oz. • Special K cereal, 1 cup • 2% milk on cereal, 4 oz. • Raisins, 1 oz.	• Black coffee, 8 oz. • Gluten-free steel cut oats, ¾ cup • Almonds, .5 oz. • Berries, 1 cup • Nutritional yeast, 2 Tbsp
Lunch	• Grilled chicken sandwich, • Large fries • Chocolate milkshake, medium (Wendy's)	• Blueberry yogurt, 6 oz. • White bread, 2 slices with 2 oz. lunch meat and 1 oz. cheese	• Large vegetable salad with chickpeas and lentils • Water infused with cucumber and lime

Snack	• 1 Clif Bar, 2.4 oz., crunchy peanut butter • Fried mozzarella sticks, 6 oz. with 1 Tbsp Ketchup • Coke- 3 (20-oz)	• 1 orange • 1 Clif Bar, 2.4 oz., • Diet Coke, 24 oz.	• Red grapes, 15 • Sunflower seeds, 1/8 cup • Water infused with lemon
Dinner	• Beef tacos, 2 • Tortilla chips, 20 with salsa • Beer, 12 oz. • Vanilla cupcake, 3.4 oz.	• Large salad with vinaigrette • Pork loin, 4 oz. • Potatoes, 2 small • Beer, 12 oz.	• Large salad with olive oil and balsamic vinegar • Roasted brussels sprouts, 1.5 cups • Wild-caught salmon, 4 oz.
Snack	• Kit Kat Bar, 1.5 oz. • Popcorn, 4 cups	• Apple, 1 • Chocolate Milkshake, medium	• Warm apple with cinnamon and nutmeg sprinkled with pecan pieces, 1 ½ cup • 73% dark chocolate, 1 oz,

Notice that in Elizabeth's beginning routine, she relied a lot on packaged and convenient foods and ate out at fast-food restaurants. Throughout the months of transitioning, she began making more of her own foods and added healthy foods she thought she could tolerate. As she refined her eating to become closer to nature, she replaced packaged foods with more whole real foods. Although she admits some enjoyment in consuming natural food and beverages, she still misses some of her favorites from the old days and occasionally indulges in them. The important term here is *occasionally*. However, she feels better now than when she ate them all the time.

Gathering Data Action Steps

Keep track of what's going in your mouth and any symptoms or cravings you may have for five days during the first week, then continually drop to one to three days a week thereafter. Use whatever tracking system is the quickest and most convenient for you. Some people like to input their eating into apps or online tracking programs, and some find it easier to write the information on paper. Others take cell phone photos of all their food and record them at the end of the day. There is no ideal way. The best way to track is the way that's easiest for you. Just do it. For a free downloadable form, visit Thenatureshift.com, where you will find a form under the Tools tab.

Throughout your record-keeping process, recognize patterns and see whether you can identify correlations between what you're eating and drinking and how you're feeling. During your record keeping, ask; What kind of impact is my food having on my health?

In the next section, "Step 2: Analyze," we'll take a deeper look at food and learn a little more about its history to help you investigate quality. I'll give you a little background on vitamins and minerals and how diseases can occur when they are removed from the diet. I'm going to share some history of a staple crop—wheat—and also talk about meat, flavorings, and sweeteners. I will attempt to help you see how the food industry plays a role in taking foods from nature and manipulating them to entice you to want more. It's my hope that when you understand more about the history of food, it will help you want to analyze it more.

STEP 2

A
Analyze the contents of the foods you eat before putting them in your body.

Chapter 6

Analyze by Learning a Food's Background

After noticing your foods, analyze their contents to be sure they are contributing positively to your body and mind.

Step 2: Analyze

   A. Analyze the ingredients on a packaged food label.

      After you are aware of the mixtures of foods you are eating from the notice step, analyze the ingredients on your packaged products. Learn about their background. By looking at the ingredients, you may find that they are safe for you to eat, or you may want to put the package back on the shelf.

   B. Analyze how close your food and beverages are to nature.

      Analyze your food to be certain it contains nutrition for your body to function at peak performance. Be certain to consume foods from farm to fork or as close to how you would find them in nature. It's helpful to visualize what your foods are doing inside your body after you swallow them. If you think a food contains sledgehammer-like additives that could wear down your cells, avoid or reduce it.

Elizabeth's "Analyze" Journey toward Eating Nature's Foods

Elizabeth started to recognize that what she was consuming was affecting her weight and health. Since she had been on the weight cycle of losing and gaining for years, she knew the convenient foods and beverages she was indulging in were problematic, but she felt stuck.

When Elizabeth started looking at the ingredients listed on her food packages and began doing internet searches to find out more about the additives, she started to wake up. She saw additives, dyes, colors, flavors, sugar, and preservatives in her packaged foods and wondered whether she should be consuming them. After analyzing the ingredients in the cookies, chips, snacks, processed meats, candy, and sodas she frequently consumed, she began to slowly take these foods out of her diet. The new knowledge of their poor quality prompted her to shift her thinking. She no longer received the same kind of pleasure while consuming them.

One day she said, "I never really enjoyed how I felt after eating hot dogs at the games on the weekends, and then I read that processed meats can cause colon cancer. I only ate hot dogs because my family liked them, and it was our tradition to eat them at the ball games. Now I know they can be dangerous for my health. I decided that I'm not going to eat them anymore. Ever. After that decision, I realized I don't want them anymore, and I look around for healthier foods to eat or bring something along. I look at them and say 'I don't eat hot dogs anymore.' It's such a freedom."

Like all of us, Elizabeth is fortunate to be living today in a time called the "Information and Experience Age" where we can get a quick answer to any food question off the internet. After gaining more education about the foods she was eating, Elizabeth shifted her food preferences and started eating more natural foods.

Throughout the upcoming Analyze chapters, it is my hope that you will gain a greater education, understanding, and background of our food supply so, like Elizabeth, you may consider eliminating foods that aren't worth the health risks and positively shift your food choices.

Lasting Effects of Poor Foods

If you transport your view back in time to the late 1800s and early 1900s, you will see people eating what they could grow, kill, trade, or buy. Since most people lived in small towns, gathering food necessitated a trip to the local township or village. Early grocery stores were more like empty rooms stocked with canned goods. If you wanted meat, you visited the local butcher; to get bread, you went to the baker and so forth.

Our ancestors couldn't look up information about food on a computer. As a matter of fact, little was known then about the science of food and how it was made up. Unfortunately, imposed by economic or cultural restraints or the inability to obtain a variety of foods, many people physically suffered the consequences of poor food choices. They became affected with diseases like beriberi, scurvy, rickets, and pellagra. Those are diseases we don't hear about today. That's because our current food supply provides the nutrients needed to prevent these diseases. However, physicians then were puzzled that beriberi, scurvy, rickets, and pellagra didn't respond to medicine. They later learned that these diseases were caused not by toxins or infections but rather by a lack of nutrients needed from food.

Back in the early twentieth century, nutrient deficiency diseases were prevalent in people who ate a lot of packaged and canned foods and little fresh foods. Alternately, the diseases disappeared when people ate a varied diet that included fresh foods. For example, pellagra, a disease that causes the three Ds—diarrhea, dementia (mental confusion), and dermatitis (blackened scaly sores on the skin)—wasn't apparent in people who ate whole wheat, potatoes, and/or certain vegetables like sweet peppers. [98] Since pellagra affected more than three million Americans, resulting in one hundred thousand annual deaths, [15] with *death* becoming the fourth *D*, there was much incentive to eradicate this disease.

Vitamin Discoveries

At the height of the pellagra outbreak, scientists knew about only carbohydrates, proteins, fats, and minerals. It wasn't until 1912 that an incredible discovery was made—food contained more nutrients than people thought. Food also contained vitamins. Vitamin A was the first in the discovery lineup, which was followed by the discovery of vitamin B_1 (thiamine), then B_2 (riboflavin), then B_3 (niacin). Can you see the pattern of how vitamins got their names?

With all the fascination about vitamins in specific foods, in the early 1930s, the surgeon general funded research to study the link between nutrition and disease. [71] This research resulted in the discovery of more vitamins and their impact on the illnesses people were facing at the time. They discovered that the remedy for curing pellagra wasn't medicine; it was the presence of niacin in food. Similarly, the cure for beriberi was found to be thiamine, for rickets it was vitamin D, for scurvy it was vitamin C, and for anemia it was iron. [34] What became clear was that nature's foods were packed full of vitamins and minerals, which gave people the right materials for their bodies to stave off nutrient-deficiency diseases. As people became educated about the importance of vitamins, these diseases decreased. The discovery of vitamins was a triumph for science. Scientists were able to nail down the chemical makeup of many vitamins and mimic them in the laboratory. This research resulted in the beginning of man-made or synthetic vitamins.

In 1937, vitamins in their synthetic form began to be manufactured and sold as vitamin supplements. When an American biochemist named Conrad Elvehjem discovered the chemical structure of niacin and showed how its use quickly improved the fiery-red dermatitis associated with pellagra, it quickly became in high demand. Niacin began to be sold in its synthetic form as nicotinic acid. Elvehjem was credited for the discovery of nicotinic acid; however, he warned that the synthetic form of all vitamins should be used only temporarily and specifically be used only for the treatment of vitamin deficiency diseases. Interestingly, Elvehjem, who later went on to be the founder and chair of the Department of Nutrition at the Harvard School of Public Health, cautioned that "vitamins should be obtained from natural foods if possible, because they are in better balance with other factors when they are taken in this form." [163] The "better balance" Elvehjem was referring to is the synergistic effects of vitamins and minerals, meaning that the phytonutrients, antioxidants, vitamins, and minerals in food function best together rather than in isolation.

Today we understand that vitamin B_3 (niacin) not only promotes skin health and prevents deficiency diseases like pellagra, which our ancestors suffered from, but also helps modern-day diseases by lowering blood cholesterol and triglycerides [93] and by supporting the nervous system. [52] However, like all vitamins and minerals, niacin is best when ingested from foods high in niacin like brown rice, chicken breasts, lentils, and seeds rather than in its synthetic supplemental form, nicotinic acid. That's because when you eat food, niacin has a chance to collaborate and work with the other phytonutrients. Vitamins and minerals are similar to humans; where we are alone, one can do little, but in a group, much can be done. Nutrients in food act in the same way to support your health.

Vitamin Sales

The early scientists who discovered vitamins and minerals would probably be amazed to see how popular supplements are today. According to a study published by the American Medical Association of more than thirty-seven thousand American adults, 52 percent use supplements daily. [79] If you are someone who relies heavily on vitamin and mineral supplements but don't eat nature's foods, consider that you're missing out on the synergistic effect of nutrients and the powerful antioxidants only nature's foods can supply. Analyze your diet and see how many times you are consuming ingredients from nature. If you aren't, *a good place to start is by eating something from nature like a vegetable or a piece of fruit every time you eat a meal or snack.*

Away with Peasant Bread

If you decide to go for it and start eating something from nature every time you eat, don't be surprised if you find yourself wanting to enliven their flavors at first. The manipulation of nature's food to help it taste better has been a coveted practice throughout history. In 1870, the steamroller mill was brought to America,[161] which took each kernel of wheat and separated it into three main parts: the bran, the germ, and the endosperm.

Here is a reveal of the anatomy, nutrients, and functions of the three parts of a wheat kernel:

1. The outer bran layer (3 percent of the kernel)
   The bran contains fiber, which aids in moving food through your digestive tract and fertilizing your gut microbiome (more on the microbiome, prebiotics, and probiotics in Chapters 10 and 19).

2. The germ (14 percent of the kernel)
   The germ contains the majority of the vitamins and minerals, including B vitamins like folate, niacin, thiamin, and vitamin B_6, which help your body function well.

3. The endosperm or middle inner section (83 percent of the kernel)
   The endosperm is the portion of the grain that makes up white flour. It contains only a trace amount of nutrients and is mostly made up of starch.

The roller mill removed the bran and germ, and crushed the endosperm, the main starchy portion of the kernel, revealing a refined, light-textured white flour. When this type of flour was mixed with fat, salt, and/or sugar, it created a blissful taste sensation. Bakers used it to make pastries, cakes, and breads; and people wanted more and more, creating a huge demand for white-floured products. Besides the light texture and taste, white flour was heavily sought after because the only people who had access to it were those who could afford it. Just like society today, people back in the late 1800s and early 1900s desired to align their lives with the wealthy class, and eating white-floured products was one way to do it.

To appease the demand, the steamroller mills went into full production, and white flour was able to be produced at a lower cost. People of every class suddenly had access to the "fancy flour." Commercially sliced bread came on the market in 1928, [112] replacing the dense "peasant bread." The general public finally had the convenience of not having to grow and reap wheat and then knead and bake their own bread. Bread became easily accessible, and bread consumption increased. The fancy flour was widely popular, sold well, and came with a fortunate unintended benefit for the manufacturers—a decrease in bugs and rodents in their storehouses. The critters learned quickly that white flour lacked the nutrients they needed to stay alive, so they moved on to seek more sustainable delicacies. [150] *Rodents didn't want white-floured products because they lacked nutrients; however, humans scrambled for them because of their light texture and pleasant taste.* (Wow, those little buggers outsmarted us humans!)

Because obesity wasn't prevalent in the United States until the 1960s, having a mill remove the fiber that slowed digestion and allowed people to eat more was an added bonus. Back then, if you were able to put on weight, you were considered affluent. Getting enough to eat was a means of survival and status. People were trying to acquire enough food to stay alive, so food quality wasn't a main consideration.

When the association was made that disease-preventing nutrients were being stripped from the wheat, the government stepped in.

Chapter 7

Analyze the Quality of Wheat

Enrichment Act

With synthetic vitamins on the market and the knowledge that they can help cure nutrient-deficiency diseases, the Food and Drug Administration (FDA) determined that specific vitamins needed to be added into foods if they had been removed. In 1942, bread began to be "enriched," which means the synthetic form of vitamin B_1 (thiamin), vitamin B_2 (riboflavin), vitamin B_3 (niacin), and iron—four of the eighteen vitamins and minerals removed from wheat— were required to be added back into the flour to prevent the nutrient-deficiency diseases mentioned earlier.

By 1943, the Enrichment Act was enacted [68] with the original purpose of ensuring strong and healthy World War II soldiers. Subsequently and thankfully, flour manufacturers were mandated to enrich all white flour with thiamin, riboflavin, niacin, and iron, saving Americans from the debilitating effects of the nutrient-deficiency diseases so prevalent at that time. The thought was that they would see no more nutrient deficiencies that caused beriberi, skin disorders, pellagra, and anemia, thereby underscoring the importance and significance of nutrition on human health. Done. But wait. More recent research revealed that they had forgotten one.

Starting in the 1940s and for many decades after, the enrichment process added thiamin, riboflavin, niacin, and iron to enrich white flour. However, with continued research, another one of the remaining fourteen vitamins not added during enrichment was discovered to prevent neonatal neural tube birth defects (NTD). The neural tube in embryonic development is the predecessor to the spinal cord and brain; when the tube doesn't close completely during fetal development, it damages these critical areas. [30]

Neural tube birth defects range from mild to severe, depending on the location. Anencephaly is the most severe of the NTDs and almost always results in death. When a person is born with an NTD, it causes lower spinal cord lesions that can cause lifelong problems including incontinence or paralysis of the legs. Research beginning in 1965 showed that the incidences of NTDs were dramatically reduced or eliminated when 400 micrograms of folate were added to the diets of pregnant women. Therefore, folic acid, the synthesized form of folate, began to be added as the fifth vitamin in the enrichment process of wheat and other processed grains like rice. Shockingly, even though vitamin B_1 (thiamin), vitamin B_2 (riboflavin), vitamin B_3 (niacin), and iron were placed in enriched products in 1948, folic acid wasn't added until 1998. [102] Therefore, during a fifty-year span, up until 1998, pregnant women who were eating enriched foods but not eating folate-rich foods or taking a folic acid supplement had a significantly higher risk of having babies born with neural tube defects.

After folic acid fortification was added to enriched foods, the number of NTDs declined 27 percent from 4,100 to 3,000 incidences. Also, the annual number of deaths from NTDs declined from an estimated 1,180 fetal deaths in the United States to 840 deaths. [102] Since the research supporting folic acid's protective attributes had been known since 1965, [60] it's distressing that such an easy fix to a devastating and fatal outcome wasn't put into action earlier. Also, if we had all simply eaten unaltered grain milled from the entire wheat kernel, these issues would have been avoided.

We can only wonder how much healthier society would be and how many fewer wheat sensitivities and allergies there would have been in the past 150 years if we had left the wheat alone and eaten unaltered flour—flour grown without some of the harmful pesticides added today and crushed straight from whole wheat kernels. How nice it would have been if nature's nutrients had never been removed in the first place. One lesson we can learn from understanding the history of food processing more is that *Mother Nature knows best how to run our bodies.* Today we know that vitamins and minerals that are important for our health like niacin, thiamin, riboflavin, iron, and folate are removed from the wheat during processing, including some lesser known important phytochemicals that protect our cells from oxidation called "phenolics" and "terpenoids." [153]

Vitamins and Minerals Stripped Today

When you leave wheat kernels intact and make flour out of them, they can give you all the nutrients you see listed in Table 4.

Table 4

Nutritional Content of Hard Red Winter Wheat Kernels

Nutritional Value in 100 Grams, 3.5 Ounces, or Approximately 3/4 Cup Dry		Dietary Reference Intakes (DRIs): Estimated Average Requirements for Female and Male Adults (19+ Years)	Percent of DRIs in 3/4 Cup Dry Wheat Kernels
Energy	327 calories	*varies	
Carbohydrates	71 g	45–65% of calories	
Sugar	0.4 g	≤ 25% of total calories	
Fiber	12.2 g	25–38 g per day	32–49%
Fat	1.5 g	20–35% of calories	
Protein	12.6 g	10–35% of calories	

Vitamins			
1. Thiamin (B$_1$)	0.38 mg	1.1–1.2 mg per day	32–34%
2. Riboflavin (B$_2$)	0.12 mg	1.1–1.3 mg per day	9–11%
3. Niacin (B$_3$)	5.46 mg	14–16 mg per day	34–40%
4. Pantothenic acid (B$_5$)	0.95 mg	5 mg per day	19%
5. Vitamin B$_6$	0.3 mg	1.3–1.7 mg per day	18–23%
6. Folate (B$_9$)	38 µg	400 µg per day	9.5%
7. Choline	31.2 mg	425–550 mg per day	6–7%
8. Vitamin E	1.01 mg	15 mg per day	7%
9. Vitamin K	1.9 µg	90–120 µg per day	1.6%
Minerals			
1. Calcium	29 mg	1000–1300 mg per day	2%
2. Iron	3.19 mg	8–18 mg per day	18–40%
3. Magnesium	126 mg	320–420 mg per day	30–40 %
4. Manganese	3.96 mg	1.8–2.3 mg per day	172–220%
5. Phosphorus	288 mg	700 mg per day	41%
6. Potassium	363 mg	2,600–3,400 mg per day	11–14%
7. Sodium	2 mg	1,500 mg per day	< 1%
8. Zinc	2.65 mg	8–11 mg per day	24–33%
9. Selenium	70.7 µg	55 µg per day	129%

Look to see what vitamins and minerals you feel are important for your individual health as you peruse the table. This table lists the nutritional value of hard red winter wheat kernels, which is the type of wheat that accounts for 70 to 80 percent of the total wheat produced in the United States today. [155]

Once you select certain vitamins and minerals you feel are important to you (which they all are) from the table, realize that after processing, most of the eighteen vitamins and minerals listed in Table 4 are removed.

Why Do They Enrich Our Wheat Today?

The unfavorable health outcomes we see today like fatty liver disease, clogged arteries, high blood pressure, weight gain, mood swings, and progression toward obesity are linked to eating too many synthetic foods. Most are made from white flour. Yet today we see more white flour than whole wheat flour being produced. White-floured products on the market outnumber whole grain products and are less expensive. It seems obvious that since we now know how important fiber, protein, fat, vitamins, and minerals are in the bran and germ, more whole wheat flour should be generated for the health benefits of society. However, this isn't the case.

Because of consumer acceptance and sales, food companies keep pumping out refined products, in which enriched flour is the main ingredient. Flour mills also reap a cost benefit. They are able to make white flour for humans to eat and then use the bran and germ (sometimes referred to as "by-products") to make food for our huge animal population to eat. The by-products go into making food for domestic animals like dogs and cats and for growing and fattening the animals on feedlots, where they are slaughtered for meat consumption. With multiple commodities to sell, the mills make more money.

Hopefully, with continued awareness of how our grain is separated today for financial gain instead of human nutrition, more people will begin to scrutinize and analyze what's going into their bodies and purchase only higher-quality, unaltered grains. Products like white-floured breads, pastas, crackers, and cookies will continue being made if there is a demand for them, so don't buy them. Instead, buy foods made from stone-ground, whole-meal, or whole wheat flour as the first ingredient. This ensures that the whole kernel is used to make the flour. Or if wheat doesn't agree with you because you have a sensitivity or allergy to gluten, gliadin, or lectin (proteins in wheat), venture into the myriad of other whole grains like buckwheat, millet, teff, barley, or bulgur. Or try consuming more legumes like soybeans, chickpeas, beans, and dried peas or their products. For example, try lentil or chickpea pasta. These nutrient-dense foods are increasingly being offered and are available at most supermarkets and online. They can enliven your taste buds, enrich your palate, and help your digestive tract work properly.

In the next chapter, we will analyze meat and seafood to help you explore some practices going on within that industry.

Chapter 8

Analyze Meat

Processed Meat: Everyone Loves Animals, so Why Do We Eat so Many of Them?

When one of our daughters was eleven, she came home from a church function with a baby chick—a live one! All the kids received one that day whether their parents knew about them or not. Before I could say no, my husband said yes. Soon our garage became filled with multiple cages, bedding, heat lamps, a feeder and a waterer. The chick (simply named Peeps) became a side hobby for our animal enthusiast daughter, and we began to inherit some of the other chicks the kids' parents said no to. Eventually a large coop showed up in our backyard, and the growing chicks were all (thankfully) moved outside.

One day a cawing noise came from one of the chicks. This noise continued to grow more and more frequent throughout the days. When we began hearing it start at four o'clock in the morning and every minute after, we knew we had a rooster in the flock. Being new at raising chickens, we had no idea what to do with a rooster, but we knew it had to go. Since some of the adults living in our household were meat-eaters, I suggested that they kill it and cook it up like in the olden days. I was met with panicked looks. No one wanted to take on the grueling task. We fortunately found a breeder to give our rooster friend to, and he ended up having a good life. However, when I went to the grocery store the next day and saw all the chicken products on the shelves, in the rotisseries, and in the freezers, it occurred to me that if all of us had to kill and cook up our own chickens or any other animal, maybe we would eat a lot fewer of them.

Obviously, when you do eat meat, eating it fresh off the bone after it has been killed and cooked is the best way. However, to keep from spoiling, meat and seafood need to be preserved. After seafood is caught, it needs to be processed or frozen soon after it comes out of the water to keep it from contamination. Therefore, you're not going to be able to consume meat, poultry, or fish straight from the land or water unless you catch it yourself and kill it, which few of us can or want to do.

Government agencies initially evaluate the preservatives and additives for safety to keep seafood, eggs, poultry, and meat fresh. The Food and Drug Administration (FDA) has the ultimate responsibility for safety, but it relies on a branch of the US Department of Agriculture (USDA), called the Food Safety and Inspection Service (FSIS), to examine and test additives for safety. The preservative nitrite is used to preserve mammalian-muscled meat, such as goat, beef, veal, pork, mutton, lamb, and poultry. Nitrates also enhance its flavor, longevity, and freshness. But the cost to your health can outweigh its convenience. As noted in Table 1 back in Chapter 3, nitrites from meats cooked at high temperatures combine with amino acids (the building blocks of proteins) in your stomach and form nitrosamines. Nitrosamines have been found to damage your DNA. [35] If you are going to eat meat, at a minimum, avoid meat that contains nitrites and nitrates. Also, be wary of celery powder, which gives you a nice dose of naturally occurring nitrate. Celery powder is a source manufacturers are increasingly using to preserve meat products, assuming that customers are on alert only for the words *nitrite* and *nitrate*.

Processed Meats Can Increase Your Cancer Risk

You may or may not be aware that some meats can increase your cancer risk. According to the 2015 report from the International Agency for Research on Cancer (IARC), the cancer agency of the World Health Organization, processed meats like hot dogs, corned beef, ham, sausages, jerky, canned meat, and bacon are classified as "carcinogenic (cancer causing) to humans." [69] Carcinogens in processed meats specifically target the stomach, colon, and rectum, contributing to stomach and colorectal cancers. Also, unprocessed red meat like pork, veal, lamb, or beef is considered "probably carcinogenic to humans." Red meat cooked at high temperatures through grilling, panfrying, or barbecuing is the most problematic because suspected carcinogens are produced more abundantly at higher heats. [69] Currently, there is no warning label on packages of meats to caution the consumer about their potential harm. However, if the negative impacts of eating processed meats keep climbing, the regulatory agencies may step in and enforce a warning label someday.

The Business of Meat

When meat is processed, it is chemically altered to increase its shelf life and promote its stability. Preservatives enhance the flavor of meat, creating an enjoyable "mouth feel." The great demand for meat has created our huge meat industry today, where animals live in feedlots to be butchered. The feedlot style of raising animals, where they live in jam-packed habitats to limit their movement, produces meat with a high-fat content and a better flavor. Because our palates crave fat, animals and seafood are raised to be as fat as possible.

The animal environmentalists have most villainized the cow because it takes the greatest resources per pound to feed. Crops like soy, legumes, silage (fermented feed sourced from barley, corn, oats, and millet), and wheat by-products, which we talked about earlier, are used for cattle feed instead of what is most natural for them to be eating—a mixture of pasture (grass), silage, and hay. [151] In comparison, cows able to roam free and graze eat considerably fewer calories per ounce than those raised on a feedlot for the slaughter market. For example, one ounce (28 g) of grass has around 28 calories, whereas the same ounce of soy, wheat, or legumes cows are fed on a feedlot has three times more calories. Equally, in the fishing industry, the same fattening techniques occur with seafood. The seafood available to us in the supermarket is mostly farmed, which means the fish are enclosed within ponds or tanks and fed high-calorie fish meal, oil, and grains.

The way animals on both land and sea are raised and slaughtered in today's traditional animal agricultural environment has caused many to become vegetarians solely on that basis.

A Solution to Decreasing Meat Consumption

Meat production is a big business, and like any business, it needs to make money to survive in a capitalist society. If we, the consumers, purchase meat raised in feedlots, we are sending a message that we want more. If we stop buying this type of meat and instead eat meat from animals that are free to roam, or skip meat altogether and replace it with more legumes, nuts, and seeds, the massive industrial factory farms would respond.

The way we currently eat meat is also detrimental to our environment. According to a 2018 sweeping analysis of the food system's impact on the environment, as published in the journal *Nature*, current animal farming methods are depleting water supplies, and polluting aquatic and terrestrial ecosystems. [141] Greenhouse gasses produced by livestock plus the effects of deforestation and water shortages are main contributors to the devastation. A suggested answer to sidestepping catastrophic environmental change is to follow a "flexitarian diet." That means the average person would eat 75 percent less beef, 90 percent less pork, and half the number of eggs, substituting animal products with more legumes, nuts, and seeds. Since eating meat products occasionally instead of frequently is better for human health, it appears that both our bodies and the earth are telling us something important about the best way to eat.

In the next chapter, Chapter 9, we will talk about the flavors in our foods. I intend to help educate you on how and why flavors are used, hoping this information will help you continue to analyze your foods.

Chapter 9

Analyze Flavor Ingredients

Flavorings: The Flavor Punch

After plants are plucked from nature, they slowly decay and lose their taste and texture. To maximize sales, food companies add chemicals and preservatives to nature's foods to enhance their flavor, consistency, and shelf life. This allows a food or beverage in a package, can, bag, bottle, or jar to be sustained until it's sold. Flavorings are so popular that roughly 90 percent of the products purchased from store shelves have added flavors in their ingredient lists, and these flavors come from chemical concoctions developed in laboratories. [87]

It's the job of the Flavor and Extract Manufacturers Association, an agency that works under the Food and Drug Administration (FDA), to assess the flavor ingredients food manufacturers use to make sure they are "generally recognized as safe" or GRAS. Once on the market, a GRAS ingredient can be used by food companies until there is enough evidence to warrant a ban and/or removal. If additives, preservatives, and flavor enhancers have passed appropriate clinical trials (which can take many years) and are found to be safe for human consumption, the FDA stamps them as GRAS. Some considerations of safety include how flavoring mixtures will be absorbed, metabolized, and excreted; and how much exposure of a compound can accumulate in a typical experimental animal's body and brain without it becoming genotoxic.

(The word *genotoxic* means any damage and/or mutations to DNA caused by a chemical agent in a food or beverage.) Genotoxicity can lead to cancer and other diseases.

The Flavor and Extract Manufacturers Association is the voice of the US flavor industry and is composed of flavor manufacturers, flavor users, flavor ingredient suppliers, and others interested in the flavoring industry. Though this association has power over flavors in theory, much of the onus to create safe products is now managed by the flavor creators and the food companies. Because the process to get a new additive onto the market previously took years to get through, in 1997 the bogged-down FDA put the responsibility on the food companies to do their own clinical trials and prove on their own that the ingredients they wanted to use to flavor their products were GRAS. [53] Although the FDA was extremely slow in approving new additives for human consumption, we consumers had some assurance that independent, unbiased scientists were reviewing, testing, and approving the safety of an additive being put in our food and beverage products. Not any longer.

Now consumers are forced to trust the food industry to police itself. If a food company's primary interest is to increase sales and not its products' safety and impact on humans, then unsafe products can be on the market until otherwise proven that they're harmful. Moreover, if dangerous additives also increase the risk of cancer, it's nearly impossible to prove that the additive from company A *caused* the cancer as opposed to the additives of companies B, C, D, or E. As the old adage says, "The fox is in charge of the henhouse."

Even if additives and preservatives pass through clinical trials and are allowed to be in the food supply, this doesn't qualify them as okay for *you*. You may be consuming foods and beverages that are safe for *others* to consume but turn out to be toxic sledgehammers in your body. Also, if you live in the United States, bear in mind that compared to other regions in the industrialized world, the United States has looser food regulations. Be sure to analyze the ingredients on the packages of any synthetic foods you buy before you consume them and be your own body's regulatory board. If you're unfamiliar with a particular ingredient, look it up to see its origin or, better yet, skip the synthetic food and replace it with a food from nature.

Scientist + Artist + Flavor Adjuster = Flavorist

Let's look at the origin of flavors put into food and beverage products. The flavorings I'm referring to are either those naturally occurring in nature or those flavorists or flavor chemists thought up. [149] A flavorist or flavor chemist has an advanced degree in areas such as biochemistry, food science, biology, and chemistry; he or she uses his or her scientific knowledge to mix precise chemicals to create flavors. The work of a flavorist is a combined field of art and science. [47] If needed, they may consult with another professional like a sensory psychologist to create products that will appeal to your emotions. It's a career field you may not be aware of because the flavoring industry sells directly to food companies and not to the public. It is a uniquely quiet multibillion-dollar industry. And because some flavors substantially improve sales and market shares for whatever company uses it, flavoring companies treat their flavors as sacrosanct.

Since experts in the flavoring field are part chemists and part artists; their scientific backgrounds mixed with their creative flair allow them to imagine new and unexpected ways to help us experience a flavor. Flavorists are so accomplished that they can fabricate flavors from nature, like the flavor of a strawberry, without actually using real strawberries. With many years of training under their belts, they have the skills needed to create unique flavors all in the hopes that when one of their flavors hits the market, you, plus the entire human population, will get hooked on it. If they can boost a product's consumption rate, sales will increase, adding significance to their work.

Flavorists refer to specific distinct smells extracted from food in nature as "volatiles," which are volatile organic compounds (VOCs) or "notes." [59] Think of all the keys on a piano. Each key is a note that can contribute to a chord. When the right keys are played in an arrangement, beautiful music ensues. The same concept applies to creating flavors. When chemical notes have been aligned in a superior organization, you taste the top note first and the bottom note last. Flavorists arrange ingredients and endeavor to impart sweet, sour, salty, bitter, or savory tastes, plus physical traits like hot and cold. These ingredients in the right mixtures create a party in your mouth.

Flavor Fantasies

Flavorists mix and match from their available GRAS chemical palette to make a seemingly unlimited number of flavor combinations. The goal of the flavoring chemist is to make sensational bursts of flavor that will give your brain a swift kick of excitement, followed immediately by a deadened sensation. This entices you to take a second bite, then a third, then a twentieth, and so on. Therefore, food and beverages are intentionally designed to compel you to consume. Food manufacturers benefit through increased sales when you buy more of their products to feel good. Nonetheless, there are big incentives to make synthetic foods as tasty as possible. The goal is to excite your taste buds and brain to eat more and buy more. Unfortunately, all this can lead to compulsive eating and even addiction. (More about addiction in Chapters 30-34).

Some flavors, like the flavor of an orange straight off a tree, created by Mother Nature, are repurposed to give products an orange flavor. Other flavors can be entirely made up, like the flavor of nacho cheese. Nacho cheese and other synthetic man-made flavors are "fantasy flavors." Food chemists and flavorists can design the flavor sensation of nacho cheese and place it directly in a chip by mixing the right notes. Here are the ingredients of a popular nacho cheese chip:

> Whole corn, vegetable oil (corn, soybean, and/or sunflower oil), salt, cheddar cheese (milk, cheese cultures, salt, enzymes, maltodextrin, whey, monosodium glutamate, buttermilk solids, Romano cheese (part skim cow's milk, cheese cultures, salt, enzymes), whey protein concentrate, onion powder, partially hydrogenated soybean and cottonseed oil, corn flour, disodium phosphate, lactose, natural and artificial flavors, dextrose, tomato powder, spices, lactic acid, artificial color (including Yellow 6, Yellow 5, Red

40), citric acid, sugar, garlic powder, red and green bell pepper powder, sodium caseinate, disodium inosinate, disodium guanylate, nonfat milk solids, whey protein isolate, corn syrup solids.

If you count all the ingredients in the chips, there are forty-two! These ingredients were carefully placed note by note to make up the nacho cheese symphony of flavors that leaves your brain wanting more.

Food companies need to protect their ingredients because there is fierce competition in the food industry for product sales. Therefore, if you try to make nacho cheese chips at home using the ingredients listed on a package, realize that the "natural and artificial flavors" in the ingredient list are a mixture of compounds from a laboratory, not from a kitchen. The notes were placed together to make up the nacho cheese flavor, and because all the chemical compounds aren't disclosed, we don't know the exact mix and quantity of notes needed to create the flavor. This unawareness prevents you and other food companies from duplicating the recipe.

Even with secrecy and strategy to create the tastiest flavor, an ideal mixture of flavors isn't enough to put a product out front as a best seller. Effort also needs to be put into design and packaging. For example, a popular snack company spent $50 million in 1994 to make one of their best-selling chips 20 percent larger and 15 percent thinner with the edges more rounded. [29] Fifty million dollars may seem like a lot of money for a company to put into research and development of a chip back in 1994, but if you consider the billions of dollars large snack food companies make in annual sales, you can see that $50 million is actually a relatively small investment.

Synthetic Food Product Labeling

As previously discussed, exotic mixtures of unnatural, chemical-based flavoring compounds in synthetic foods need to find a way to lure you, the consumer, into eating them. Food companies use nutrition-related buzzwords like "natural," "gluten-free," "organic," or "whole grain" to mislead you into thinking a product is somehow good for you, creating a false sense that the food or beverage is healthy. [33] For example, here are the ingredients from a package labeled "Natural" Jelly Beans: sugar, corn syrup, cornstarch, dextrose, fruit juice concentrates (apple, lemon, tangerine, peach, strawberry, blueberry, grape, cherry, pomegranate), citric acid, pectin, sodium citrate, natural coloring (fruit & vegetable extracts, beta carotene, annatto, turmeric, riboflavin, saffron, caramel color, titanium dioxide), natural flavors, ascorbic acid, beeswax, carnauba wax, vanilla, confectioner's glaze, salt.

By law, ingredients on a package need to be listed in descending order; therefore, when you analyze the ingredient list above, note the order of ingredients. The first two ingredients in Natural Jelly Beans are sweeteners from both sugar and corn syrup. The third and fourth ingredients are cornstarch and another sugar, dextrose, followed by fruit juice from concentrate. Next on the list are preservatives and binders from citric acid, pectin, and sodium citrate; then there are a variety of "natural colors" followed by "natural flavors" and more preservatives, binders, and flavoring agents. The word *natural* on the product is a very loose term. The only ingredients actually from nature, listed after the sugars and cornstarch, are fruit juices from concentrate. As you analyze your foods, don't be swayed by marketing words like "natural" but instead read ingredient lists for clarification of a product's quality. These "natural" jelly beans are highly processed and have only a smidgen of nature in them. After reading the label, I personally wouldn't eat or recommend them.

More About "Natural" and "Artificial" Flavorings

The flavoring industry must follow criteria the FDA established that define the proper use of a "natural flavor" or "artificial flavor." A natural flavor is something derived from some kind of plant or animal matter, where the function is to create flavor, not give it nutrition. As discussed earlier with the "natural" jelly beans, this definition is counterintuitive. As consumers, we tend to think "natural" means something is from nature and is healthy and good for us. In reality "natural flavoring" means that the original compounds used to make a product taste better were derived from something in nature like a spice, fruit, vegetable, yeast, herb, bark, root, or leaf. It can also come from meat, seafood, poultry, eggs, dairy products, or fermentation products.

One example of a compound that can be termed a "natural flavor" is an organic compound called 4-hydroxy-2,5-dimethyl-3-furanone or Furaneol. [108] This compound comes straight from strawberries. If it is used in a product to get a strawberry or fruit flavor, it can be listed as a "natural flavor" on the ingredient list because it is sourced from the strawberry. This is the case even though the strawberry-flavored compound derived from the fruit is so minimal that it contains no nutritional value. However, if a flavorist instead uses a strawberry-flavored compound that was originally created in a laboratory called ethyl methylphenylglycidate—big words here, I know—to create the strawberry or fruit flavoring in a product, it would be classified as an "artificial flavor." Both compounds can give a product like gum, strawberry ice cream, and candy a fruity or strawberry flavor, but if one works better than the other in a flavoring mix, the superior compound will be used for obvious commercial reasons.

By law, the chemical names 4-hydroxy-2,5-dimethyl-3-furanone or ethyl methylphenylglycidate aren't required to be listed on a label. As long as these ingredients fall onto the GRAS approval list, they can be dumped into the category of "natural or artificial flavor." What's more, the natural or artificial flavors you see on an ingredient list are typically a mixture of many compounds, not a single chemical. They can range from a few to more than fifty compounds in their flavoring mixes. However, you have no idea what or how many (five, fifty, one hundred?) are sequenced to make the right flavor. It's alarming that such a complexity of compounds with names we can't pronounce can go straight into our bodies and brains as potential sledgehammers, and we as a society are typically unaware that they have been strategically and carefully placed in our food products. Again, the food and beverage manufacturers are allowed to determine the safety of these chemicals without third-party validation.

One final point about "natural flavors" is the looseness of the term *natural*, which requires some—albeit limited—association with living organisms. But interestingly, the living organisms used to create natural flavors aren't required to be edible. Rather, they could be from leaves, tree bark, or the anal castor sac of a beaver. Not kidding, castoreum is the name of a compound from the castor sac of beavers, with all the implications associated with the word *anal*. The beaver excretes this brown liquid castor sac substance to mark its territory, as dogs do. It has an appealing vanilla-like fragrance and has been on the FDA's GRAS list since 1965. [19] It has been used in vanilla-flavored products, but of course, it's not listed on any ingredient list because, like all naturally sourced chemicals, it is disguised as a "natural flavor." Fortunately, castoreum is cumbersome, expensive, and difficult to obtain since there are only so many male beavers in the world. The important takeaway from this is that whether the flavor is natural or artificial, the true ingredient mixture is a *secret,* and you may be consuming things that are, well, disgusting.

Citrus Beverage versus an Orange

To continue our analysis of ingredients, let's take a look at a popular citrus beverage. Here are the ingredients: water, high fructose corn syrup and less than 2 percent of concentrated juices (apple, orange), ascorbic acid (vitamin c), alpha tocopherol acetate (vitamin E), vitamin A palmitate, citric acid, natural flavors, pectin, canola oil, modified corn starch, Yellow 5, Yellow 6, sucralose, sucrose acetate isobutyrate, sodium citrate, potassium sorbate and sodium hexametaphosphate (preservatives), and calcium disodium EDTA (to protect color).

The only ingredient recognizable as citrus in the ingredient list is concentrated orange juice, which is less than 2 percent of the product. That means water, high-fructose corn syrup, and the other ingredients on the long list of additives are 98 percent of the citrus beverage.

In contrast, the ingredient list of an orange straight off a tree is the following: vitamin C, (as found in many citrus fruits), which protects your immune system, heart, eyes, and skin; beta-carotene to assist in vision; [76] thiamin, which plays a key role in nerve, muscle, and heart function and as previously mentioned—the vitamin needed to prevent beriberi; [31] choline for methylation, which helps your body regulate memory, muscle control, and mood; [169] folate, which assists your DNA in cell division, preventing neural tube defects along with megaloblastic anemia; [23] potassium, which helps you maintain your fluid volume, muscle contraction, and nerve signaling; [146] fiber, which helps fight cancer, lower both blood sugar and blood cholesterol levels, and helps your food flow through your digestive system; [89] and citrus flavones (a type of flavonoid), which aids in memory and elevates your moods.

By the way, the majority of an orange's flavones are found in the white part, called the "pith," so peeling and eating an orange helps you reap the majority of the orange's antioxidants. Unfortunately, the most nourishing parts of an orange are removed when it is made into juice, and no nutrients are found when it is processed and used in the flavored citrus drink listed above.

What's more, by consuming an orange instead of drinking a sugar-ladened citrus drink, you receive both choline and folate—the same nutrients (from Chapter 4) the pregnant mice were fed that gave their pups methyl groups and shut off obesity, cancer, and diabetic genes. To follow a path of wellness, make a change from foods and beverages full of artificial ingredients and replace them with those nature provides.

Sugar, Fat, and Salt Trio Bliss—Give Me More!

Just like the flavorings from synthetic foods can cause a drug-like boom in the brain, so can sugar, fat, and salt. In food laboratories, when the explosion to the brain is sourced from sugar, it is referred to as the "bliss point" or the amount of sugar that makes the product most enjoyable and hard to resist. [128] When the richness of the fat is just right, it is called a good "mouthfeel;" [43] and when the salt mixture is ideal, it's said to be "optimized." [4] Sugar, fat, and salt in the right combinations will bring short-lived rewards to the brain. When at least two of the sugar, fat, and salt trio are heightened and in the right combinations, your brain's pleasure-seeking centers are triggered. If you combine the pleasurable sensations you receive with the neurotransmitter dopamine, your brain will remember the food or beverage and will send you to find the delicacy again. (More on dopamine in Chapters 16-18). Dopamine sends chemical messages between nerve cells and helps to motivate you to learn new things. [12] With eating and drinking, dopamine helps you to estimate whether it's worthwhile to pay attention to the food you just consumed. This awareness allows you to decide whether you want to eat the food again. If you decide to consume a food or beverage padded with sugar, fat, and/or salt again and again, you are basically saying to food manufacturers, "Please continue selling this product."

In the next chapter, we will discover more about your tongue's taste receptors and dive deeper into high-intensity sweeteners—more ingredients that stimulate your brain.

Chapter 10

Analyze Sweeteners

Your Tongue's Indulgence with High-Intensity Sweeteners

High-intensity sweeteners, previously called "artificial sweeteners," stimulate your tongue's sweet taste receptors and give your brain the illusion that you are indulging in something sweet. As of the time of this writing, there are six approved high-intensity sweeteners in the United States: acesulfame potassium (Ace-K), advantame, aspartame, neotame, saccharin, and sucralose. Stevia from the leaves of the stevia rebaudiana plant, luo han guo (monk fruit) from the siraitia grosvenorii plant, and allulose from wheat, corn, figs, and raisins are approved sweeteners that originated from plants but are heavily processed to be made into granules. There are also sweeteners in your foods called "sugar alcohols." Sugar alcohols you may see on an ingredient list include sorbitol, mannitol, xylitol, maltitol, maltitol syrup, lactitol, erythritol, isomalt, and hydrogenated starch hydrolysates. Sugar alcohols are only partially absorbed [96] by your body and therefore don't give you as many calories as if you were eating sucrose or granulated table sugar but have a laxative effect that can cause gas and bloating.

Then and Now: Decades of Frozen Sweetened Chemicals

Companies use a blend of high-intensity sweeteners to find the "bliss point." For example, ice cream companies devised a master mix of ingredients to make ice crystals within ice cream taste as sweet and creamy as possible. They also know that to maximize sales, cartons of ice cream can only sit in a store's freezer for two to three months unopened until they need to be purchased. Some frozen desserts in the grocery store have a long list of ingredients that have been used for decades. Marketing a product like ice cream with the label "no sugar added" helps to increase sales because it is attractive to those hoping to eat healthier. But high-intensity sweeteners used as an alternative to sugar stimulate your hunger in the same way. Here is what you will see on a 2022 version of a "no sugar added" ice cream. All the sweeteners in the ice cream are in italics.

> Ingredients: non-fat milk, cream, fudge swirl (*maltitol syrup***, water, cocoa processed with alkali, modified corn starch, *maltitol***, salt, natural flavor, xanthan gum, *sucralose*, nonfat dry milk), *maltitol syrup***, peanut butter cups [chocolaty coating (coconut oil, *lactitol***, *maltitol***, cocoa processed with alkali, soy lecithin, vanilla extract), peanut butter (peanuts, salt)], maltodextrin, *polydextrose***, glycerin, natural flavor, milk minerals concentrate, cellulose gum, mono and diglycerides, salt, *sorbitol***, guar gum, *sucralose (Splenda® brand)*, carrageenan, citric acid, vitamin a palmitate, annatto color, *acesulfame potassium*. contains: milk, peanut and soy ingredients.

On the label are these words: "** Sensitive individuals may experience a laxative effect from excess consumption of this ingredient."

In comparison, here is an older version of a "no sugar added" ice cream in a similar flavor from the same company dated 20 years ago in 2002: Ingredients: non-fat milk, cream, chocolate fudge swirl (*maltitol syrup**, water, cocoa processed with alkali*, modified corn starch, salt, *aspartame*, natural flavor, xanthan gum), polydextrose*, *sorbitol**, maltodextrin, cocoa processed with alkali*, whey protein, mono and diglycerides, cellulose gum, cellulose gel, carrageenan, *Sunett® acesulfame potassium*, vitamin A palmitate, *aspartame*. contains: milk and soy ingredients.

On the label are these same words: "* Sensitive individuals may experience a laxative effect from excess consumption of this ingredient."

If you read both ingredient lists carefully, you will see that although they are labeled as "no sugar added," there are five to nine sweeteners in each ingredient list. "No sugar added" means only no sucrose or table sugar added, but the "no sugar added" and "sugar-free" claims can still have a high percentage of sweeteners in them as long as those sweeteners aren't sucrose. Because Americans like things sweet, high-intensity sweeteners and sugar alcohols have made their way into our products with a vengeance. The types of sweeteners added to products have changed over the years (in part due to public acceptance), but the amount has either remained the same or increased. You will notice that listed twice on the 2002 ice cream label was aspartame. This sweetener was omitted in the 2022 version, but the newer version had nine total sugar alcohols and artificial sugars in the ingredient list. The 2002 ice cream had only five. Sadly, the changes in the ice cream over time seem to have made it actually more toxic to your system and not healthier. Yet since the sweetness in ice cream makes it taste so good and your tongue seeks the sweet, creamy flavor, those who produce ice cream know they have a steady clientele despite the ingredients.

Your Microbiome

If you continually indulge in foods with an abundance of high-intensity sweeteners like the "no sugar added" ice cream listed above, you are interrupting the workers inside your body that run your immune system. You have an extremely large biocenosis of microbes living inside you called your "gut microbiome." (More on your microbiome in Chapter 19). Studies show that high-intensity sweeteners negatively impact the balance of this vast ecosystem of microbes within, leaving you susceptible to illnesses. [21] Your microbiome can be impacted by what you eat, breathe, or what may come in through your nose, eyes, genitals—or through bites or wounds that breach your skin.

Your microbiome is simply all the microbes that live in and on your body with their genetic material. Although the exact number is not concurred, scientists believe your human body hosts about one hundred trillion microbes, and the majority of these live in either your colon or large intestines. [13] Your microbiome contains live, unimaginably small beneficial bacteria, viruses, protozoa, fungi, and helminths. [41] To give you an idea of their size (because they are so small), most bacteria are usually measured in microns. Viruses, being even smaller, are measured in nanometers. To illustrate these measurements, consider the size of the period at the end of this sentence. The period is about 350 microns or 350,000 nanometers in diameter. To see infectious bacteria that could cause pneumonia, you would have to magnify the bacteria to 350,000 times its actual size just to get it to the size of the period. To make a virus the size of a period, it would have to be magnified 26,250,000 times. [41] It's amazing to me that through modern imagery and science we have the ability to magnify the details of what a nanoscopic virus looks like up close and understand how they function. Studies have shown that high-intensity sweeteners reduce the diversity of your good microbes, [91] creating an environment where fewer beneficial microbes are present and intestinal inflammation can occur. This condition permits illnesses to set in. If you always seem to catch whatever is going around and find that you get sick a lot, cut out high-intensity sweeteners to build up your good microbes.

Prebiotics and High-Intensity Sweeteners

One of the most essential nutritional agents you can eat to help your microbiome is fiber. Fiber in nature's foods can construct healthy colonies, whereas high-intensity sweeteners can destroy them. Fiber is referred to as a prebiotic because it acts like a fertilizer to feed, nurture, and build colonies of healthy microbes throughout your digestive tract. Once microbes come in, the high-fiber (prebiotic) substances from complex carbohydrate plant-based foods go to work to strengthen your healthy colonies of microbes.

You have good microbes in your gut to fight off harmful invaders that attack your immune system. Over time as you eat more fiber from nature's foods and decrease additives like high-intensity sweeteners, you will increase your healthy microbial population and help your brain and body function at full throttle.

Probiotics

Probiotics work with prebiotics in a reciprocal relationship that support one another in defending your body against invaders. Probiotics from nature's foods come from fermented foods where the carbohydrates and sugars are transformed by bacteria to stabilize and prevent the food from spoiling. In the time before refrigeration, this process was necessary to make produce nonperishable. The probiotic foods you may be most familiar with are yogurt, kefir, sauerkraut, and kimchi. People who regularly eat these foods get an added boost of healthy microbes that assist their immune system, making probiotic foods a valuable asset to the body.

Chapter 11

Analyze Food Advertising

Food Quality and Advertising

When analyzing the foods you eat, be wary of those that are highly advertised. Marketers are trained to push out products in hopes that you, the consumer, will buy them and get hooked. With few exceptions, there is an inverse relationship between the amount of money that goes into advertising a food product and the quality of the food or beverage.

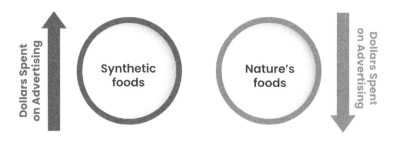

For instance, in the United States, $1.5 billion was spent on food and candy advertising from 2018 to 2020. [143] Conversely, farmers growing nature's foods don't spend nearly that kind of money on advertising.

Due to the obesity epidemic in all age-groups, including children, adolescents, and adults in the United States, some leaders within the food industry are questioning the ethics of marketing synthetic foods to consumers and are seeking ways to better promote fruits and vegetables. For example, companies that predominantly grow a single kind of vegetable like carrots want to increase their product lines to make a wider variety of fresh products available to consumers. Others are willing to provide consumers with prepackaged grab-and-go carrots or sugar-snapped peas. There are also leaders in the food industry who want to increase transparency about their food products. They recognize that some consumers are surprised to discover how much sugar, fat, and salt are in their foods and are looking for healthier alternatives. For the benefit of our health, let's hope that the pendulum will continue to swing toward food companies offering and marketing healthier foods.

Send a Message: I'll Buy Natural, Real Food

Food companies have to make money and are sometimes stuck if they formulate healthier versions of their products that don't sell. If they have to compromise their profits and obligations to their shareholders, they will find a way to make a product taste amazing, no matter what they have to add to it. It's the basic law of supply and demand. *The one power you have as a consumer is to stop buying synthetic foods and start purchasing and eating more of nature's foods.* As a consumer, your wallet is your voice. When you buy and eat fresh foods because you *want them*, you are speaking to the food companies that you like what they have to offer. Nature's foods that are fresh and convenient are increasingly being added to the market. The more money you spend on these products, the more the food industry will adjust to meet the demand.

Note: If you have gotten this far in your reading and haven't already felt galvanized to start your own grain fields, vegetable gardens, and fruit tree orchards, you can begin your journey toward healthier eating by analyzing the quality of your foods and choosing to purchase and eat fresh unaltered foods. It's my hope that if you're not there already, you will go back to eating more of what is grown outdoors and use your purchasing power to show that you don't want synthetic ingredients in your food. As you follow the nature steps, you will notice your palate changing, and over time you will be able to say with confidence, "I crave nature."

Chapter 12

Analyze Produce

If you are ready to start eating more produce or if you're just venturing out to give it a try, below are some tips on what to look for to analyze fruits and vegetables. To receive the highest-quality, best-tasting, and safest produce, choose one or two tips to focus on when you shop.

- **In Season**. Fruits and vegetables contain their peak nutritional content when they are in season and are harvested closer to the peak of freshness. They also taste better than those that spend a lot of time in shipping or in a warehouse. Type "fruits and vegetables in season" into your internet browser to find resources on what produce is in season in your area. Many books also share information about which foods are in season when.

- **Frozen**. To get most of the same nutrients as fresh, try frozen. Fruits and vegetables are usually picked and flash-frozen when they are at their peak. Consuming frozen produce is the next best thing to eating fresh.

- **Farmers markets**. The produce available at your local farmers market usually gets harvested right before it's available for purchase. Market produce is picked closer to the time you eat it compared to what you find in a grocery store. It also tastes amazing.

- **Color**. To get the best produce, look for deep, rich colors. Nature's foods contain vibrant reds, yellows, oranges, greens, whites, purples, and more. When you pick out your fruits and vegetables, be certain that their colors are rich and beautiful. Color is an indicator of higher antioxidant levels and ripeness.

- **Stems**. Many fruits and vegetables will indicate that they are at peak ripeness when they feel a little softer around the stem. Also look for green stems instead of brown ones.

- **Smell**. Ripe fruits and vegetables will give off a noticeable fragrance. You want to smell a tomato scent when you put a ripe tomato near your nose. Notice the sweetness of strawberries when you pick up a carton of them. When looking for the best cantaloupe, push down where the vine was attached. If it's somewhat soft and has a sweet, fragrant smell, it's ready.

- **Washing**. The best way to preserve the fruits and vegetables you have at home is to wash them right before you plan to eat them.

- **Residue Removal**. When crops are sprayed with pesticides, whether they are organic or conventional crops, the residue remains on the produce's surface. A good way to remove pesticide residue is to mix a little sodium bicarbonate (baking soda), about one teaspoon per two cups of water, and wash the surface. One 2017 study found that baking soda was more effective than bleach or tap water alone at removing residue. [166]

Chapter 13

Analyze Summary, Recommendations, and Action Steps

My "Analyze" Experience

After analyzing the foods I frequently ate, I realized I consumed a lot of packaged synthetic foods and beverages. Even though I tried to include more produce, I was influenced by and ate what my family and friends wanted to eat. In my refrigerator, I stocked sweetened beverages like soda and juice, ground beef, lunch meat, sour cream, and a little produce like guacamole, apples, and carrots. My pantry was filled with white-floured pasta and tortillas, jars of spaghetti sauce, cans of soup, white rice, sweetened cereals, chips, cookies, and crackers. On a typical evening after looking in my refrigerator and pantry to get something to eat, I often made a burrito with a white-floured tortilla, ground beef, cheddar cheese, canned refried beans, guacamole, and sour cream. Pretty good, huh? It was my standard go-to dinner. While writing this book, I decided to nutritionally break down the burrito I frequently ate to see exactly what went into my body. Here is a table of the breakdown:

Food	Calories	Protein	Carbohydrate	Fat	Sat. Fat	Trans Fat	Sodium	Fiber	Phytonutrients/ Antioxidants, ORAC value*
8-inch tortilla	146	3.8 g	25.3 g	3.1 g	0.4 g	0 g	249 mg	0 g	0
2 oz of ground beef	186	4 g	0 g	8.4 g	3.2 g	0.6 g	37.6 mg	0 g	0
1/4 cup of cheddar cheese	106	10 g	0.4 g	11 g	7 g	0 g	205 mg	0 g	0
1/4 cup canned of refried beans	54	11 g	9 g	1 g	0.2 g	0 g	267 mg	3 g	904 µ mol TE/100 g
1 oz of guacamole	164	2 g	8 g	15 g	2.4 g	0 g	65 mg	5 g	1922 µ mol TE/100 g
2 Tbsp of sour cream	46	0.8 g	2.6 g	4.8 g	2.8 g	0 g	19 mg	0 g	0
Total	702	31.6 g	45.3 g	43.3 g	16 g	0.6 g	842.6 mg	8 g	2826 µ mol TE/100 g

*Oxygen Radical Absorbance Capacity or ORAC Test

The last column on the chart contains the Oxygen Radical Absorbance Capacity (ORAC) value, which measures the antioxidant count of food. The ORAC test is performed by placing food in a test tube along with certain molecules that are vulnerable to oxidation and generate free radical activity. The less free radical damage to the food, the higher the antioxidant capacity.

There are some limitations with the ORAC test, so the numbers in the table are for informational use rather than hard scientific evidence that one food is superior to another. For instance, the ORAC score doesn't measure synergistic effects between nutrients. In the body, processes of growth and repair are typically linked. One process activates or affects another. Therefore, nutrients in your food typically work better in combination with other nutrients. For example, one study of two antioxidants, quercetin (found mainly in apples, onions, and berries) and catechins (found mainly in apples, green tea, and purple grapes), discovered that together these two antioxidants help to stop platelet clumping, which leads to blood clots and heart attacks. [122] Neither had the same effect when used alone. Since apples are on both lists, the next time you eat an apple, think about how the antioxidants are helping your bloodstream function better. And, yes, eat the peel. A good portion of quercetin and catechins are found there.

I found that when I started analyzing the quality of the foods I was consuming, I started to make more conscious decisions on what foods I would eat based on what was in the food. *I wanted to find tasteful, affordable, easy-to-prepare foods and beverages that lacked a lot of additives and were as close to nature as possible.* It initially took me a while to sort through the products on the market to find ones that met my criteria. This was and is an ongoing process because new products are frequently being added to the marketplace. I found myself becoming fascinated by all the selections available, and I began scouring labels of new merchandise or studying the produce for something new to try.

Today I think I've narrowed down a good mixture of foods for myself and my family that give us variety while providing our taste buds with new adventures. I try to avoid products that have any kind of "flavorings" in them, but that's tricky. They are in the majority of packaged processed food products on the market. Therefore, I cook and eat as close to unprocessed foods as possible. However, even with my best intention to eat healthily, I've been surprised to find "natural flavors" snuck into health food products like protein powders, meatless products, tempeh, and ready-to-eat lentils, to name a few.

Today, instead of making the previous burrito, I would eat something like grilled red peppers, baked wild salmon, and a side of quinoa. Here is a table of this breakdown:

Food	Calories	Protein	Carbohydrate	Fat	Sat. Fat	Trans Fat	Sodium	Fiber	Phytonutrients/ Antioxidants, ORAC value *
2 cups of grilled red peppers	92	3.8 g	18 g	.8 g	0 g	0 g	12 mg	6 g	847 μ mol TE/100 g

1 tsp olive oil	40	0 g	0 g	4.5 g	0.6 g	0 g	0.1 mg	0 g	372 µ mol TE/100 g
1/2 cup quinoa	114	4 g	20 g	2 g	0 g	0 g	5 mg	2 g	3200 µ mol TE/100 g
4 oz salmon	232	25 g	0 g	14 g	2.8 g	0 g	68 mg	0 g	30 µ mol TE/100 g
Total	478	32.8 g	38 g	21.3 g	3.4 g	0 g	85.2 g	8 g	4449 µ mol TE/100 g

Burrito

Total	702	31.6 g	45.3 g	43.3 g	16 g	0.6 g	842.6 mg	8 g	2826 µ mol TE/100 g

In comparison to the burrito, the salmon dinner gave me a better overall nutrient profile. After analyzing the burrito I frequently ate, I realized that for the 702 calories it cost me, I could do better. At the time, I was a typical sedentary woman, who needed 1,200 calories per day to maintain my basic metabolic requirements, plus an extra 400 or so calories for movement, which totaled around 1,600. (More on individual calorie needs in Chapter 23.) The 702-calorie burrito cost me almost half of the total calories my body needed for the entire day and wasn't worth it. Moreover, this one burrito contained a whopping 842.6 milligrams of sodium, which is over one-third of the 2300 milligrams of sodium my body needed.

The pepper, salmon, and quinoa dinner improved my calorie, protein, carbohydrate, fat, sodium, and antioxidant count. The burrito had an ORAC score of 2,826—mostly from the guacamole, whereas the peppers, salmon, and quinoa had 4,449. I was excited that I was bringing in a healthier dose of nutrients and more antioxidants to protect my cells and boost my immunities. Also, I discovered that if I cooked the peppers, quinoa, and salmon just right, they were delicious.

Analyze Recommendations

Analyzing your foods doesn't require you to construct a chart to discover all the calories, proteins, carbs, sodium, and ORAC scores. Rather, simply be curious about what you're eating and decide whether you're consuming good-quality foods. Also, if you're eating something from a package, look at the ingredients. Determine which ingredients you recognize.

The first step - "Notice"— recommends that you put awareness into what you are eating and keep a food diary. This valuable tool helps you to gather data on what's going in your body. Once you know what's going in, analyze the origin of the food and how it is contributing to your body and health. Analyze how you feel every time you eat certain foods. If you feel bloated, headachy, less energetic, or just unpleasant after eating, especially from a synthetic, processed food, replace it with nature's food. If you think it's helping to repair and nurture your body, choose it again. If you analyze the ingredients of a packaged food and observe that it's full of unwanted additives, try a food from nature instead. Gradually increase the quality of foods you consume while decreasing low-quality synthetic foods.

Experiment with nature's foods. Prepare a large salad with a variety of colorful vegetables or a medley of roasted vegetables. You may be at the point where eating vegetables seems daunting, but I promise you can do it, and your body *wants* you to do it.

Here are some basic recipes you can use to help you start eating more vegetables. One is a salad with homemade vinaigrette; the other is a grilled vegetable recipe.

Green Salad with Vinaigrette
Prep Time: 5–10 minutes

Ingredients:
4 cups mixed spring greens
1/2 cup shredded carrots
1 cup grape tomatoes
1 red onion, chopped or sliced thin
1 cup berries

Dressing
1/4 cup white wine or balsamic vinegar
3 tablespoons fresh lemon juice (or the juice of 1 lemon)
1 clove garlic, minced
2 tablespoons fresh basil or 1 teaspoon dried basil or 1 teaspoon ground cumin
1 teaspoon locally made honey or 1 teaspoon monk fruit
1 teaspoon Dijon mustard
1/2 teaspoon sea salt
1/4 teaspoon black pepper
2 tablespoons parsley, minced
3 green onions, minced
1/4 cup extra-virgin olive oil

Preparation:
1. Place the vinegar, lemon juice, garlic, mustard, honey, sea salt, and pepper in a blender and blend.
2. Add the fresh chopped parsley and onion. Blend.
3. Add oil and blend (if possible, slowly stream in olive oil through an opening in the top of the blender).
4. Season with salt and pepper.
5. Toss the greens, vegetables, and berries with the dressing and serve at room temperature.

Yield: 8 servings, 1 serving = 1 and 1/2 tablespoons

Nutritional Information:
Per serving: 79 calories, 0 grams protein, 4 grams carbohydrate, 7 grams fat, .5 grams fiber
*If you notice, this recipe is only 79 calories per serving—and it is filling! If you're looking to lose weight or keep the weight off, eating nature's foods is the way to do it.

Grilled Vegetables   Prep Time: 10 minutes   Cook Time: 12 minutes
Set grill to medium/high or heat oven to 350 degrees.

Ingredients:
1 medium zucchini or 1 yellow crookneck squash with ends removed, sliced in half lengthwise, cut into 1/2-inch pieces
1 eggplant, ends removed, cut into 1/2-inch pieces
1 red onion, peeled, ends removed, cut into eighths
3 sweet peppers (red, yellow, and/or orange), stem and seeds removed, sliced into eighths
1 carton mushrooms (8 ounces), halved
1–2 tablespoons olive oil
Salt and pepper to taste
Optional: 2 tablespoons fresh herbs (like basil, oregano, parsley, rosemary, or thyme), minced

Preparation:
1. Wash and dry vegetables. Cut according to the directions above. Set aside mushrooms.
2. Place vegetables on 24-by-17-1/2-inch piece of heavy-duty foil for outdoor grilling or on two 13-by-18 baking sheets if roasting in the oven.
3. Drizzle vegetables lightly with olive oil.
4. Sprinkle fresh herbs, salt, and pepper over vegetables.
5. If grilling, bring opposite edges of foil together, leave a little space for steam to build. Grill, stirring every 2–3 minutes for 10 minutes. Add mushrooms. Continue grilling an additional 10 minutes until lightly charred and tender.
6. If roasting, place baking sheets into a preheated oven. Stir every 2–3 minutes for 10 minutes. Add mushrooms. Continue roasting an additional 10 minutes or until tender.

Yield: 8 servings (1 cup each)
Nutritional Information: Per serving: *50 calories, 3 grams protein, 5 grams carbohydrates, 2 grams fat, 5 grams fiber
*Again, here. Only 50 calories per serving. And you will be satiated!

When you have either the salad or grilled vegetables ready to eat, here's a mindful analysis exercise I invite you to do:

> Reinforce your food choices by analyzing what's on your fork. Visualize your digestive tract becoming nourished by all the wonderful healing agents the vegetables will provide. This may seem unusual, but it is critical and very effective in your mental progress toward healthy eating. Visualization is powerful. Try to see where those vegetables originated and how they were grown in nature. Ponder how the rain and sun allowed the vegetables on your fork to grow to maturity. Imagine all the elements from the earth working together to form and create those vegetables. Tucked inside the vegetables on your fork are thousands of nutrients ready to enter your body and provide your trillions of cells with energy and healing agents. Just think—with every bite, you are restoring your body with antioxidants that protect your cells from damage. Remind yourself that *eating nature's foods is a form of self-compassion and self-preservation that only you can give to your body.* Remind yourself, "I'm worth it!"

Believe it or not, if you approach your eating with the mindful analysis above, your palate will eventually shift, and you may find that even if you didn't initially like vegetables, you will begin to accept them and one day enjoy their flavors. If you're still skeptical, realize that it's sometimes normal to initially reject nature's foods, especially vegetables. I've noticed it takes at least six taste encounters and attempts at new foods like vegetables before the brain accepts them as palatable. That's no empirical study, just my observation with my family and patients over the years. So give new vegetables at least six separate attempts before you give them up.

When you substitute synthetic foods with nature's food, slowly but surely you will begin to desire their flavors more. If you never give nature's food a try, you will lose out on filling yourself up with nutrients and fiber and mending any needed cellular damage created by the sledgehammer effect of free radicals.

Action Steps for Step 2: Analyze

A. Analyze the Ingredients on a Packaged Food Label

As a rule of thumb, the longer the list of ingredients, the fewer the nutrients. Find and consume products with ingredients you can pronounce.

Look out for artificial and natural flavorings, or both. If these flavorings are present, realize the food or beverage has compounds that are "generally recognized as safe" (GRAS) but are from sources that aren't fully disclosed and are potentially undesirable, dangerous to your health, or both.

B. Analyze How Close Your Food and Beverages Are to Nature

Determine how far a food or beverage is from nature. If the food you want to consume has gone through many processing steps, then vital nutrients needed to nourish your body have been removed. Consider another food choice.

Visualize what your food and beverages are doing inside your body when you consume them. If they are causing negative symptoms, avoid or reduce them.

The following worksheet is a guide to help you analyze the ingredients in packaged or processed foods. Write them down here:

Ingredients of Processed Food #1	Do You Recognize the Name of This Ingredient?	Do You Think This Ingredient Is Helpful or Potentially Harmful to Your Body?	Do You Want to Continue Consuming This Ingredient?

Ingredients of Processed Food #2	Do You Recognize the Name of This Ingredient?	Do You Think This Ingredient Is Helpful or Potentially Harmful to Your Body?	Do You Want to Continue Consuming This Ingredient?

In "Step 3: Train," we'll look at the brain and memories. We'll explore how shifting cravings is possible. We'll take a look at how brain chemicals can impact food choices, and we'll review taste and smell. The chapter concludes with ideas to lower your stress and provide you with a script to meditate in a way specifically designed to help you visualize your ideal self. We will learn more about what drives your preset automatic habits and how you can train your brain to make the shift toward nature.

STEP 3

T
Train your brain to form new positive connections with nature's foods.

Chapter 14

Train Journey

After noticing and analyzing the foods you're eating, train your mind to crave them.

Step 3: Train

A. Train Your Thoughts and Visualize Your Future Self Enjoying Nature's Foods

Once you decide to consume nature's foods, see yourself mentally as if you're already there. If you can imagine yourself eating and drinking real food from nature, then you can achieve it through your actions. Change your thoughts toward nature's foods by starting with "I am," then end with words that define you as if you are already living in your identified desired state of being. To help with this change process, write down and draw a motivational phrase, which is discussed later in this chapter.

B. Practice

Learning to seek foods from nature takes practice. There are nerve signals that need training. For long-term success, gradually swap in nature's foods as you decrease synthetic foods. Slowly but surely you will begin to desire and ultimately crave nature's flavors.

C. Meditate and Practice Mindfulness and to Manage Stress

Stress hormones can interrupt your ability to rewire your brain. Thoughts like *Should I consume this or not?* are not activated during stress. To cope with life's stressors, practice stress-management techniques or begin a meditation practice with tips listed at the end of this chapter.

Elizabeth's "Train" Journey toward Eating Nature's Foods

Elizabeth sat in my office and plunged her hand into her purse. She retrieved two well-worn pictures: one was of a large house, the other of a sports car. As she showed me their images, she told me she had carried these photos around for over fifteen years. In a nostalgic tone, she said, "When I was younger, I always wanted to live in a house like this, and I always wanted to drive this kind of car [referring to her photos]. And guess what? Now I do!"

As we examined how effective this imagery was for her, I asked, "Now why don't you use the same visualization practice you used to obtain your house and car to get the body you want?"

She put my suggestion to action. To shift her brain into seeing herself as she wanted to be, Elizabeth started putting up photos of herself around the house back when she had been at a comfortable weight. Seeing the slimmer version of her body throughout her household gave her mind a positive focal point, which replaced her current image. Owning the fact that she was going back to her leaner self gave her a resolve to swap in healthy foods. Little did she know that she was training her brain to eat in a way that would give her the body she wanted.

Why Should You Crave Nature's Foods?

Like Elizabeth, are you seeing yourself as you want to be? Does your logical mind tell you that you need to change your eating and drinking habits? If your last doctor's appointment was a clean bill of health no matter your lifestyle, you're probably content with your current state of eating and living because in whatever you're doing, you're getting away with it. *If, however, your health has deteriorated and you're feeling the effects of disease—low energy, more fat on your body, and/or a general feeling of malaise—you have good reasons to shift your focus and create new habits.* Maybe you are scared that if you don't change, you won't live as long. Or you would love to break free from your current state, but the diets you've tried before didn't work, and you don't want more deprivation in your life. Some of my clients get stuck thinking that if they just eat "diet" foods until they feel better or lose weight, then they can go back to eating synthetic foods in the long run. Realize there is another direction you can go. There's a different journey to acquiring better health and longevity than what you are used to. Believe you can override memories and train your brain to eventually begin craving foods that help you feel and look better. Throughout the next few chapters, we will explore how your brain is influenced by what you eat and what strategies you can use to train your brain to eat from nature.

Chapter 15

Train New Memories

Eating Influencer #1: Classical Conditioning

To examine how your brain is governed by what you eat, let's first look at one of the most famous experiments with food and conditioning—Pavlov's dog experiment. You may have heard of it already, but if not, here are some details. In the early 1900s, the Russian physiologist Ivan Pavlov conducted an experiment that shed light on food and conditioning and is still relevant today. [129] Pavlov put out food and simultaneously rang a bell to see what the dogs in his experiment would do. When the food was present and the bell sounded, the dogs salivated. They associated the sound of the bell with a food reward. Pavlov then took the food away and just sounded the bell. Even in the absence of food, the animals salivated at the mere sound of the bell. By combining bell ringing with food, the two events became connected in the dogs' brains. Today, more than one hundred years later, the same associations Pavlov saw with his dogs remain true in humans. For example, think of what food comes to mind with the mention of one of these events:

- Watching a movie in a theater
- Sitting at a baseball game
- Being at a birthday party
- Celebrating Valentine's Day

- Grilling on the Fourth of July
- Enjoying Thanksgiving

Now, here are the foods and beverages you may have associated with each event:

- Watching a movie in a theater: popcorn
- Sitting at a baseball game: hot dogs, beer
- Being at a birthday party: chips, cake, ice cream, cookies
- Celebrating Valentine's Day: chocolate, wine
- Grilling on the Fourth of July: barbecue ribs, watermelon
- Enjoying Thanksgiving: stuffing, pumpkin pie

When you are present at one of the events listed above, you may begin salivating for some or all of the familiar foods and beverages mentioned. Maybe even just an invitation to one of these events like a birthday party or a wedding will excite a craving for cake and ice cream.

Some people get stuck when they have programmed their minds to respond to food cues. For example, let's suppose you're watching TV and see two commercials. One shows cheese melting on a burger, and in the other, a cold beer is being poured into a glass (the bell rings), and you begin to salivate. Even if you don't actively go out and immediately eat a cheeseburger and drink a beer, you respond by salivating. Marketers who are clearly familiar with food cues and conditioning will advertise tempting foods because they know cravings happen after people see and hear them.

Besides the sight of food, cravings are also ignited by other senses like smell, touch, or sound. For example, maybe you gave up bread for good but find yourself salivating for it after smelling the wafting scent of it baking. Or you want to eat the fried chicken you touched with your hands after licking the juices off your fingers, or you may find yourself desiring a soda after hearing the crisp, bright sound of it being poured. *Your senses along with the force of advertisements, the availability of synthetic foods, and for some, the need to suppress unwanted emotions, cause an internal compulsion to consume.* After you give in to a craving, your brain forms a memory that what you devoured was delicious, and it wants you to repeat the indulgence. Don't despair, however. Over time as you start to form new memories with nature's foods, old links become weakened, and new ones become strengthened.

Eating Influencer #2: Memory Trap

Many people find that despite their best intentions to change their eating to dine on roasted vegetables, tempeh, quinoa, and drink only a glass of water, they end up going back to quick favorites like whipping up a package of mac and cheese, dried noodles, or something that brought them comfort during childhood. Memories of familiar foods, beverages, and circumstances are stored throughout the brain. With our current understanding of the human brain, we don't have a quick and easy way to stop memories and cravings for specific foods. Memories of eating food that gave your brain a buzz or a dose of nostalgia are hard to escape and are reinforced every time you consume familiar comfort foods. Also, if you expect to one day completely forget about the old foods you once indulged in, realize it's not that easy. When new memories are formed, they will override but not permanently erase the old ones. [129]

The amount of attention you pay to the foods you are eating also tie into memory formation. Let's say you are about to eat a food you are completely unfamiliar with for the first time. You will, no doubt, be highly observant and maybe even a little hesitant. That's because your brain is wondering whether the food or beverage is safe. Once you have tried it multiple times and have established that it isn't poisonous or a threat to your survival, you have the freedom to process additional thoughts and perform other tasks while eating. You relax into this new eating and drinking routine, and over time you are free without thought to eat as a secondary action to whatever else you are doing. Once established as safe, eating can happen subconsciously and automatically while you are watching TV, driving, or browsing the internet. And because your brain is so clever, once you link a chosen activity with food or drink, an association and memory are formed between these two events. The activity becomes a stimulus or prompt to eat or drink, and your neurological pathways go into automatic piloting. This allows you to grab familiar foods, beverages, or both, and eat mindlessly and unconsciously while your brain is busily engaged in something else like a favorite TV show.

Eating Influencer #3: Childhood Messages

Another way your brain may be influenced by food is by childhood messages. The experiences programmed into your food preferences can be affected by how food was presented to you when you were a child. If food was offered as a contingency—like you were required to eat all the peas on your plate if you wanted a cookie—then you learned that you had to get through the undesirable peas before you were able to be rewarded with a cookie. What you were really being told was that there would be "no joy until you suffered through those vegetables."

If this is how you were raised, this kind of training actually enhanced your desire for the forbidden, desirable cookie and simultaneously added to your aversion to peas. During this time, you formed an opinion that peas were to be rejected because there was something inherently wrong with them, or you most likely found yourself rebelling against whoever was keeping you from the cookie. These memories linger into adulthood and subsequently cause the same reactions to foods and authorities that are encoded earlier in life. If this scenario is true for you, work on reintroducing the contingency foods slowly and give them a fresh start.

Eating Influencer #4: Prohibition

In my experience, most people succeed in following healthy eating recommendations for a time but don't maintain those behaviors for more than a few months. Honestly, how does it feel when you're told that to be healthy or feel good you have to give up favorite foods, which contain sugar, dairy, gluten, carbs, and lectins, or have to give up whatever is on a "no-no list" forever?

There are many reasons why you don't want to give up your favorite substances, but for now let's say *you don't want to change because if the thrill you receive when you eat or drink is taken away, there is nothing else to replace it*. If this is the case, lists of "don't do this" are mentally unsustainable. Nobody enjoys lists of prohibited foods and beverages, especially if they are some of the few excitements or pleasures during the day. Prohibition makes people feel spiteful and rebellious.

If you can identify with one or all of the eating influencers and find yourself constantly consuming synthetic foods, over time you build up a tolerance to them, which causes you to require more and more to feel satisfied. Slowly but surely, your desire for them intensifies. *Americans have built up such a tolerance to synthetic foods that alarmingly each person in the United States consumes on average 10.6 grams (42.5 teaspoons) of sugar, 79 grams of fat, and 3,400 milligrams of salt per day.* [113] For Americans to change their taste preferences, there needs to be a shift in the palate. This shift can begin with you!

Eating Influencer #5: Repetition

Another way we unconsciously eat is through memories formed from repetition. When you eat or drink throughout the day, repeating your actions rebuild past experiences. This reconstruction influences your reactions. Since memories are processed and stored as either short-term or long-term ones, every time you eat something, whether it be candy or cauliflower, a memory is reprocessed and brought into long-term storage. Therefore, repetitive behaviors become habits stored in your long-term memory. For example, if you snack on salty or sweet foods like crackers or cookies at night, you create a long-term memory that programs you to eat these foods every evening. Through repetition snacking becomes a learned skill. You are eventually able to "perform" the snacking skill with exact precision and without thought because snacking has become automatic. Kind of like scratching an itch.

The good news is, you can override your long-term memories to prevent synthetic foods from duping you into craving more. There are structural and functional changes that happen in your brain that allow new memories of eating healthy foods to go from fragile to stable. [1] Just as the repetitive practice and consumption of eating synthetic foods can increase the desire to eat more of them, the practice of eating real foods can do the same.

Chapter 16 gives insights on unconscious and habitual eating and reaffirms that the best way to tackle lists of prohibited foods and beverages is to start building a list of nature's foods to enjoy. Over time you will establish a palate for them, and you will override old memories of synthetic foods and replace them instead with memories of real, healthy food. Positive memories of nature's foods will reignite your desire to eat them more.

Chapter 16

Train Your Brain to Retrain

Habituation

One of my daughters has four kids, each two years apart. After she had her fourth child, I stayed with her for several weeks to help her get settled in. One night after putting the kids to bed, my four-year-old grandson called from his bedroom. He couldn't go to sleep because we had forgotten to brush his teeth. I escorted him to the bathroom, supervised him while brushing, and then tucked him back in. Everything was better, and he was ready to fall asleep. My grandson was already following the simplest ingrained memory process called "habituation."

When you were a kid, you may have been taught manners such as saying "please" and "thank you" and doing basic hygiene that turned into adult habits like washing your hands before you eat or, like my grandson, brushing your teeth before bed. Through years of repetition, these ingrained manners became habits. In science, much of habit learning is referred to as nondeclarative, implicit, reflex, or unconscious learning. [21] Whether you realize it or not, the way you eat regularly and the tastes you enjoy are unconscious skills developed from hours and hours of practice. The taste of the foods you habitually eat is the result of the brain's efficient use of its energy and resources. The reason your brain forms habits when you perform the same routine over and over again is to allow your mind to create space for new learning.

The repetitive process of eating a food you highly desire so you can feel good is an example of habituation. Let's say your go-to food to elevate your moods is cake (if cake doesn't suit you, replace the word *cake* in the upcoming section with your favorite food or beverage). Eating cake to combat negative emotions is a learned process that develops over time and doesn't happen when you eat a piece of cake for the first time.

Let's break down the cake-eating process (or highly desired food): Physiologically, when you bite into a mouthful of cake, your blood sugar rises quickly from the sugar. This triggers neurotransmitters and hormones called "endorphins" which give your brain a kick of excitement and pleasure that can overrule any other emotion. Endorphins continue after your first bite since one mouthful isn't enough to fuel your entire body. The euphoric feelings you experience from the sugar rush can also be intensified if you are in a happy setting like a party or a wedding. As more sugar from the cake enters your mouth, an enzyme called salivary amylase goes into accelerated action to break down the sugar into glucose (blood sugar) molecules. Glucose gets absorbed directly into your bloodstream, and your bloodstream funnels the sugar straight to your brain. Although an average brain weighs only three pounds, it requires about 20 percent of all the calories you consume in a day so your brain has a voracious appetite for quick calories in the form of sugar. [126] When glucose hits your brain in a huge load, like from a piece of cake, your brain is assured that calories are plentiful, and it wants more. Gradually the pleasure-seeking endorphins diminish, and you receive signals to stop eating. [95, 158]

Your brain is hungry and demanding. The release of another neurotransmitter dopamine stimulates your brain to continue the same pleasure-seeking activity of eating cake and gives you the green light to take another bite and another and another. Dopamine plays a role in multiple brain functions like feeling pleasure, thinking, planning, and finding things interesting. [159] All these brain functions drive you toward your food choices. Dopamine assists your cake-eating experience by arousing you with the motivation to eat more and more of the cake, assuring you that there's a reward with each bite.

Another neurotransmitter that is activated during the process of cake eating is serotonin. Serotonin affects your cognitive processes, allowing you to act or not act. It enables you to make a connection as to the value of eating another bite of cake. Serotonin also stabilizes your mood. [25] After you've had enough cake, dopamine will teach your brain to remember the experience, and serotonin will rate cake eating as a high-value experience. Your reward systems will temporarily be tapped out, but the memory of eating the cake will be pleasant, and the dopamine and serotonin on board will busily store the experience in your memory. Your brain will register the experience and confirm that "eating cake is pleasurable." When you repeat the cake-eating event to feel good, you are forming a habit. Over time if you eat cake every time you need a pick-me-up, your brain will program the neurons to eat it automatically and unconsciously anytime you want a perk. It's the process of habituation working at its finest.

Spike-Timing-Dependent Plasticity

Another theory that explains how the brain gets into patterns of eating is spike-timing-dependent plasticity (STDP). This theory posits that neurons in your brain that support specific thought processes, like when you crave a certain food, can be increased if the connections between the neurons are strengthened. [138] In STDP, the timing of the pre- and postsynaptic space or junction between the nerves determines the strength. This means that the more you think the same thoughts, the stronger and sturdier your thought connections become. For example, *I feel sad, so I'll eat tortilla chips to help me be happy* is a thought that may occur during a time of sadness. Therefore, subsequent episodes of feeling sad trigger you to respond with your previously programmed way of acting and lead you to forage for your favorite chips. Over time the combination of being sad and then robotically eating chips for happiness is embedded in your neurons, making it an *automatic* habit. Concurrently, after you program habitual eating of tortilla chips into your automatic wiring, you form fond memories, which then give your brain an added boost of nostalgia when you see, smell, or taste the chips. However, change happens in this same network if you replace the chips with crunchy vegetables—especially beets, celery, or carrots, which contain natural sources of sodium to replace the tortilla chips. You are able to rewire your brain and increase the strength of the connections between feeling sad and automatically looking for a baggie of carrots instead of tortilla chips.

Chapter 17

Train Your Habits

Habits: Smell, Walk, Eat, Repeat

As previously noted, consuming nature's foods or synthetic foods becomes a trained skill. The area of your brain called your "motor cortex" is the place where nerve impulses initiate voluntary muscular activity. [148] In this area of the brain, you recruit the same neurons over and over again when you repeat an action. Because eating and drinking are a continual cycle of habits that repeat themselves over and over again, they first require a prompt that is built into your sight, smell, taste, sound, and touch sensory receptors. For example, a prompt could be walking into a mall, smelling cinnamon rolls, and getting diverted from why you went to the mall in the first place. The wafting smell of cinnamon rolls may trigger a happy or calming memory, so you buy one, eat it, and then temporarily feel better. The important word here is *temporarily*.

Also, if you frequently go to a mall and walk straight to a cinnamon roll shop, surprisingly the nerves in your legs become conditioned to walk that route. You also activate previously programmed motor neurons from the subsequent times you went to get cinnamon rolls. It becomes easier to go directly to your usual cinnamon roll eatery because like a robot, you are programmed to walk there. Pretty soon, buying and eating a cinnamon roll becomes automatically associated with shopping at the mall. Conversely, just like programming yourself to get cinnamon rolls, you can condition yourself the other way. For example, if you routinely visit a local farmers market every Saturday to pick up fresh produce for the week, your motor neurons will instinctively remind you when you wake up on a Saturday morning that it's time to go to the farmers market.

Prompt, Eat/Drink, Reward

Before you eat, your brain receives a stimulus or prompt to eat or drink. Think of your prompts and which of your emotions or senses excite you to eat or drink the most. Perhaps it's physical hunger, emotion, boredom, or watching TV. When you receive a prompt to eat, as previously described, automatic nerve firing activates your prompt, eat/drink, or reward cycle, which repeats over and over again as shown in Figure 3-A.

Figure 3-A

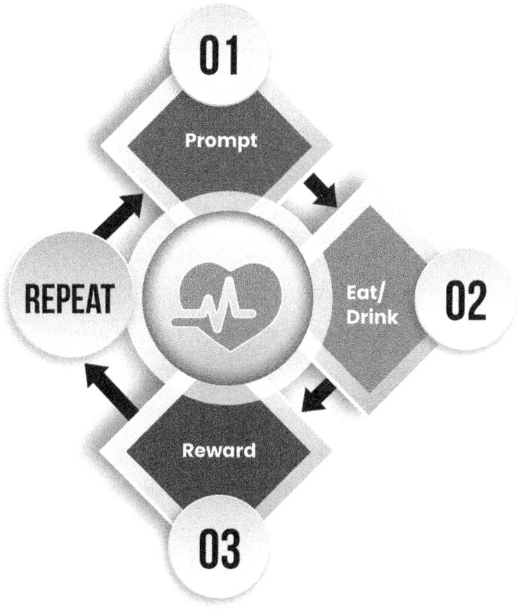

Pay attention to your prompts and what drives you to eat or drink. Emotions like anger, sadness, fear, joy, and boredom or senses like sight, smell, taste, sound, or touch can be primary motivators to eat or drink. One of my clients trying to lose weight was having a difficult time resisting food. Her family frequently left packaged foods out all over the kitchen and didn't realize the sight of food was my client's primary downfall and motivator to consume. It wasn't until she moved out and was away from her family that she learned that when tempting foods were out of sight, there was no more prompt or temptation to eat. Problem solved. My client was able to lose weight and maintain the weight loss.

Three Prompts That Lure You toward Synthetic Foods

1. **Survival Messages**. Prompts from programmed survival messages are difficult to undo. For example, once you've sampled high-calorie foods that entice your senses, there is a lure toward choosing them again and again. Part of the reason you are so drawn to foods high in calories is that these foods reassure your brain that calorie storage in the form of fat is abundant, and eating them ensures that there will be a stockpile of energy to pull from when food is scarce. Since you're programmed for survival, your brain prompts you to find and eat high-calorie foods over and over again. However, besides putting weight on you, high-calorie synthetic foods that lack vitamins, minerals, and antioxidants can actually lead to malnutrition. Consequently, people who experience this kind of malnutrition feel prompted to continue eating an overabundance of synthetic foods, hoping their bodies will receive nutrients, even at the expense of being overweight.
2. **Dopamine**. Another internal prompt for eating is the amount of dopamine your brain secretes. As noted earlier, dopamine is a neurotransmitter that helps with learning and motivation, [12] and it activates your reward circuits. Research shows that dopamine receptors are decreased in individuals who are overweight. Due to this deficiency, overweight individuals may be triggered to

overeat to compensate for the decreased activation of reward circuits. [159] In other words, carrying around extra body weight can prompt you to eat more in the hopes that you'll get more dopamine through consuming food.

3. **Safe Foods**. A third prompt your brain may give you to indulge is the internal assumption that synthetic foods are safe. Your brain recognizes synthetic foods as being safe because ultra-processed, synthetic foods have a longer shelf life than fresh foods. Thereby, your brain knows its chances of biting into a moldy piece of candy are significantly less than biting into a moldy piece of fruit. For safety purposes, your brain logically understands that you can eat candy or other synthetic foods without fear of being poisoned. This logic may prompt you to consume synthetic foods over nature's foods.

Once you identify your primary prompt to eat a synthetic food, whether it's one of the three just mentioned, or your own, work toward replacing it with a food from nature. One adjustment that has worked well for my clients is clearing their visual environment away from tempting foods. Instead of having synthetic foods lying on your kitchen counter, clear them away and simultaneously stock nature's foods on your counter and in your refrigerator. When you open your refrigerator, have previously prepped fruits, veggies, or salads with lentils, beans, edamame soybeans, or quinoa, ready to grab and eat. Healthy foods that are convenient and accessible will make it easier for you to eat nature's foods. You can find recipes from my meal plan at Thenatureshift.com.

How You Learn to Like the Foods You Eat

Figure 3-B shows, in a simplified form, my interpretation of how the process of learning what foods and beverages you want to consume works. From the time you were born until now, you have had to pay attention to hunger signals. Hunger is a physical prompt that leads you to eat something. When the food is in your mouth, you may decide that it's bad, bitter, moldy, harmful, or disgusting, in which case you stop eating the food. Or you decide the food or beverage is appetizing, in which case you continue to eat it. Both synthetic foods and nature's foods are flavorful, but they hit your taste receptors differently. As we established earlier, synthetic foods are cleverly designed to give your taste receptors a punch and your brain a quick dose of neurotransmitters and hormones, whereas the flavors in nature's foods are more subtle and brilliant. Repeatedly entertaining nature's foods on your palate allows you to adopt new, implicit habits for nature's foods.

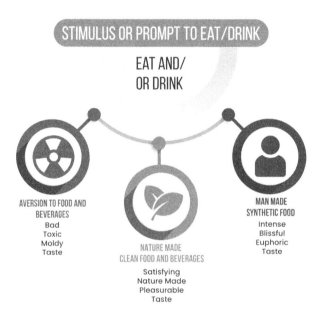

Practice Causes Attraction

There's nothing better for training your brain and body to enjoy nature's foods than the practice of it. The more time you spend eating real foods, the more you develop a taste for them. Since *what you practice causes the strength of the nerves in your brain to grow stronger*, [1] your brain becomes more attracted to whatever you routinely eat. This means that the more you practice eating nature's foods, the more you will be attracted to eating them, and the more you will receive powerful antioxidants to regenerate positive memories. Practice, practice, practice.

As you nourish your brain with healthy foods, your brain will assist you in craving them. Habitually *wanting* and craving nature's foods take application.

Please keep in mind that learning to seek and eat foods from nature isn't an overnight process. There are new nerve signals that need training. When healthy foods are introduced to your palate for the first time, you may reject them. If so, don't give up. As noted before, in my observation it takes six attempts (on average) before your brain will accept new foods. To desire new healthy flavors permanently and for long-term success, it's best to gradually swap in nature's foods rather than to exchange everything at once.

Chapter 18

Train Your Taste Buds

Detecting Taste

If I were to slice up a ripe mango and persimmon and let you choose which to eat, why would you choose one over the other? It's a short answer—taste. Even though they are similar in nutrients, your decision to eat either depends on your past experiences. If you are hungry and you have tasted one of the fruits and not the other, you will most likely go for the familiar one. The main reason most people choose what food to eat is taste. As you introduce more real foods, understand that it takes time to train or retrain your taste receptors to enjoy them. Your tongue is covered in receptors that detect five basic tastes: sweet, sour, salty, bitter, and umami (savory). Your tongue taste receptors contain on average of two thousand to four thousand taste buds with microscopic hairs called "microvilli." [67] Many of my clients get into a rut of consuming the same foods repeatedly and are then surprised when they start getting tired of them. When you eat the same foods repeatedly, your brain gives you signals that it's time to move on. Even if you eat a favorite food every day, it eventually gets boring. We call this "taste fatigue." Most people eventually get sick of repetitive foods and want something new. When this happens to you, utilize your body's need to eat an assortment of foods. Take the opportunity to unhinge from eating synthetic foods and start to branch out into the wide variety of foods nature provides. And as a bonus, you will receive the important nutrients your body needs.

Besides your tongue, you surprisingly have taste receptors in other parts of your body. For example, you have taste receptors in your digestive tract (gut), pancreas, and lungs. Here are the ways these distal taste receptors help you learn to like nature's foods:

- **Gut Taste Receptors**—The gut taste receptors in the digestive tract work with your body's microbes to inform the brain when digestive functions need assistance. Due to the massive amounts of microbes living in your gut, current research has discovered that there is competition for nutritional resources to keep certain strains of microbes alive. [61] Because it's survival of the fittest in the gut, when you crave a specific food, it may be because your gut taste receptors and microbes are pestering your brain to find that exact food.

  If you're stuck craving synthetic foods and want to change, one good thing to keep in mind is that your microbial communities can alter and assist your change process. Within 24 hours of eating healthier, your microbiome will begin to shift and create more bacteria that prefer nature's foods. [140] Therefore, your gut taste receptors help you decide and choose what to eat. Researchers in this area are increasing their understanding of how microbial manipulation and gut taste receptors either contribute to good health by helping you crave nature's foods or add to major health problems. When the gut fosters cravings for synthetic foods, this can lead to diabetes, obesity, and diseases of the gut.

- **Pancreas Taste Receptors**—Another organ you may be less familiar with that contains taste receptors is your pancreas. Your pancreas is a gland organ that secretes hormones and enzymes to help you digest your food. After you eat, your food is broken down into blood sugar (glucose), and your pancreas releases the hormone insulin to take glucose from your bloodstream into your cells. Research shows that your pancreas has taste receptors. Insulin is found to be secreted from the pancreas as soon as the pancreatic taste bud cells *sense* a sweet taste. [134] As you eat more natural foods, your sugar consumption naturally decreases, and your pancreas will be less taxed. This helps you crave less sugar and assists your enzymes to do their jobs better.

- **Lung Taste Receptors**—One more organ that contains taste receptors that need addressing is your lungs. The taste receptors in your lungs detect bitterness in plant-based foods. Researchers have discovered that bitter aspects of plant foods can have a medicinal effect on your airways. [18] Some bitter foods include arugula, broccoli, cabbage, citrus peel, cranberries, dandelion greens, kale, and radishes. The next time you eat one of these foods, think about how wonderful they are for your lungs.

As your taste receptors work together to detect taste, remember, the trick to loving food from nature is to eventually change your receptors so they *want* healthier options. It all begins when you start eating more natural foods.

Your Nose and Taste

Another major player in the taste of food and your ability to change the flavors you enjoy is your nose. Your nose contains fifty million olfactory receptor cells [135] that allow you to detect a myriad of smells. These neurons send information to your amygdala and hippocampus—two known memory storage areas in the brain. Your nose works in tandem with your tongue to detect the flavor of food. Actually, 80 percent of taste happens by smell. In fact, without smell, our food wouldn't taste as pleasant. Think of the last time your nose was stuffy; didn't food taste bland?

Your nose houses one of the most important change agents for craving nature, your olfactory nerve cells. Nerve cells are generally fixed, which means you don't grow them; however, your olfactory sensory nerve cells *do* replicate. These cells actually die, recycle regularly, and replenish themselves from neuronal precursor or stem cells every forty to sixty days. [135] This renewal process is significant because if *olfactory nerve cells can regenerate, that means you can rewire your taste preferences to crave nature's foods.* Your olfactory nerves are major players in your craving shift.

When odor and taste are combined, information is sent to the primal, dopamine-releasing part of your brain, called your anterior insula, [133] where emotions, instead of cognition, occur. This area of your brain creates the perception of flavor, explaining why the mere aroma of certain foods and beverages can stimulate powerful emotional memories. One memory that forms for me whenever I smell apple cider is being at a cider mill when I was a child. When I was four years old, my family moved from California to Michigan. The first house we lived in had several apple trees in the backyard. Each fall when the trees were full of apples, my dad picked them, put them in crates, and loaded them up, along with us kids, into our VW van. We went to the local cider mill. I remember watching the apples we had picked move up a slanted conveyor belt to a grinder, where juice was squeezed from the apples. We walked out with several gallons of cider our family drank all winter long. The smell was amazing. To this day, whenever I smell apple cider, it takes me back to that time during my childhood.

Chapter 19

Train Your Gut

How Your Digestive Tract Affects Your Brain

Researchers have discovered that what comes into your digestive tract (a.k.a. "gut") affects your brain. This concept may seem commonplace today, but studying the complex microbiome is relatively new to the scientific field. Words like *prebiotic* and *probiotic* weren't used when I was a young dietitian in the 1990s. It wasn't until 2001 that sequencing technology and other applications allowed scientists to discover and explore the microbiome and examine the gut-brain-microbiome connection. [124]

This little description may help you connect the dots between your gut and brain:

To describe how your gut microbiome affects your brain, consider that your digestive tract is an incredibly long passageway that runs through your body with openings at each end. As you know, your brain is where your executive functions occur, and directly below your brain is your mouth—the front door where food is delivered. Food that enters the mouth is swallowed and passed into your digestive tract, which drops the food deep inside your body. Alongside your digestive tract runs your vagus nerve, which works with your hormones, immune system, and a host of other complex functions to take information from deep inside your body all the way back up to your brain and vice versa.

[17] Your vagus nerve acts as an informant to help your brain coordinate a response against any invasion that may be caused by disease-causing microbes called "pathogens." If a food, beverage, or anything else you swallow contains pathogens, as a first line of defense, inflammation in the form of swelling, heat, or pain sets in. Your brain does its executive job of activating an army of workers (your immune system) to help prevent the spread of the invaders into your bloodstream, where they can travel to other locations in your body and do more harm.

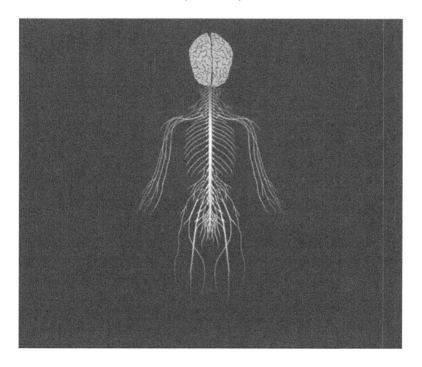

Your gut talks to your brain more than your brain talks to your gut. Actually, 80 to 90 percent of your vagus nerve fibers are called *"afferent* nerve fibers" because they go from your digestive tract to your brain. These fibers inform your brain when inflammation is present and also regulate your energy metabolism to let you know when you're hungry or full. [17] The other 10 to 20 percent of your vagus nerve fibers are called *"efferent* fibers" because they travel from your brain to your digestive tract. Their main job is to regulate the number of digestive enzymes needed to digest your food. The fact that 80 to 90 percent of your vagus nerve fibers go from your gut to your brain shows that the foods in your digestive tract are heavy hitters in brain function. It's important to keep your vagus nerve in good working order by eating the right foods and keeping yourself at a good weight. If you have extra fat stored in your upper body, called "visceral body fat," you can compress your vagus nerve, resulting in the loss of signals received from vagal afferents. You can lose the ability to regulate your appetite and become satiated (feel full), which in turn can cause your appetite and eating to increase. [14]

Brain Shift

Your cravings can and do shift, and it's possible for your brain to desire healthier foods and beverages. *Your brain and gut, working in tandem, can habitually anticipate and desire healthy foods.* The process begins by adjusting your thoughts toward eating nature's foods. The more you think about foods that will nurture your brain and body, the more you will look for these foods, and the stronger and sturdier these thought connections will become. You can train your brain to desire healthy plant-based foods by shifting your focus. Maybe you've already experienced this brain training without realizing it. Just think about a food or beverage you used to enjoy consuming but later switched. A client of mine shared an experience that illustrates how tastes can change.

She recently traveled back to the place where she had grown up in Texas. Her family, as usual, made her favorite childhood chicken fried steak. Before her visit home, this client had been working with me for over a year and had cleaned up her eating. Initially, she was looking forward to eating the chicken fried steak she had missed from her childhood, but in reality she was no longer used to the grease. She exclaimed, "It made me sick." Instead of trying the food again and again to see whether she would get used to it, she ruled it out and decided she was done with chicken fried steak. Walking away was easy for my client since there was no pleasure in a food she used to enjoy. This change wouldn't have happened so quickly without the time she had first put into eating nature's foods for a period. She noticed that her body reacted negatively to the fried food and decided it wasn't worth eating anymore.

Your desire for certain foods also changes when they go out of trend or style. When this happens, your brain shifts away from them. Depending on how old you are, you may or may not have eaten Jell-O. For those unfamiliar, this shiny, jiggly, colorful, and sometimes fluffy gelatin was very popular in the United States from the 1950s to the 1980s. Most social gatherings included some sort of Jell-O mixed with an endless variety of canned or fresh fruit, vegetables, whipped cream, marshmallows, and/or sour cream. If you find it served anywhere today (perhaps at a funeral), you may feel like you stepped back in time. Jell-O is a sweet food you might have developed a taste for back in the day. Now that it's scarce, if you once had a preference for it then, chances are you don't have the same desire now. Because it's no longer widely available, you may have trained your brain to seek another food.

Just like your brain shifts away from foods or beverages you stop consuming, you can start foraging for new flavors, even if the initial taste isn't exactly pleasant. One of my clients is a wine collector. He has a wine cellar and has been all over the world, collecting red wines. However, my client admits that red wine was an acquired taste. He didn't start off loving the taste of red wine the first time he tried it. Eventually, after encountering multiple taste samples and experiencing the multisensory stimuli wine gave him, my client began to desire its taste. The same can be true for nature's foods like vegetables. You may first dislike all or some kinds of vegetables but eventually tolerate them, accept them, and then finally enjoy them. For most, liking nature's foods takes time and encouragement.

Here's another example of brain training: Let's say you frequently eat lunch at the same place every day but change your usual bacon double cheeseburger and fries for a grilled chicken salad. While eating your salad in the same place where you normally had the bacon double cheeseburger and fries, you start remembering how pleasurable your familiar foods were. You knew you enjoyed eating them, but with your new understanding of the healing properties of nature's foods, pleasure now kicks in from the salad. There's a different excitement and reward in your brain for eating the salad—you know you are nourishing your body, which encourages you to keep eating the salad. At this point, you are programming new memories that give you a distinct kind of pleasure, similar to the way you feel after you do something that lifts your soul. These new memories override old memories. As you repeat eating the salad instead of the bacon double cheeseburger and fries, you may be surprised to discover that even though one type of food was enjoyable at one point in your life, new healthier foods are giving you a similar perk.

Read on to the next chapter and discover how stress affects your cravings.

Chapter 20

Train Yourself to Undo Stress

Stress: The Greenlight for Eating Mindlessly

What has been shared about your brain so far is based on normal or usual brain function. When you are under stress, however, your brain fires differently. Stress causes problems in your brain. [99] When high levels of stress hormones circulate, the neurons firing in your prefrontal cortex become dampened. [100]

The prefrontal cortex, the area of your brain where reasoning and executive processes occur, [168] helps you weigh the pros and cons of what to eat and drink. It also helps you understand the reasoning behind why you eat certain foods. The prefrontal cortex lends a hand in helping you make good decisions or rationalize bad ones. And most importantly, it can assist you in adjusting your eating and drinking habits to be able to achieve your health and weight-loss goals.

From an evolutionary standpoint, the prefrontal cortex is the newest part of the brain, and research has discovered that it is affected more by your environment than by your genetics. [83] This area of the brain is the sensible, cognitive region you rely on to make changes—like when you decide to take action after you have received news from the doctor that your health is deteriorating or start to do something about your weight after seeing your body in a full-length mirror.

When your executor temporarily goes quiet during stress, there is no function to tell you what to do, so your more primitive brain areas kick in, and you cycle into nondeclarative, implicit reflexes or unconscious ways of coping. In other words, stress stalls the reasonable side of your brain and leads you back to automatic consumption of previously programmed foods (which usually means synthetic foods). *If you are programmed to eat synthetic foods to relieve stress, your stressed brain will resort to mindlessly consuming them to survive. That way your brain can focus on strategies to combat your stressor(s) instead of spending time planning new foods to eat.* Fortunately, once programmed differently, the prefrontal cortex can also remind you to choose nature's foods instead of synthetic ones.

A good example of the impact previously programmed foods can have on your brain is an experience a client of mine shared. This client was experiencing incredible job stress and simultaneously decided to give up a lifelong nightly ritual of eating ice cream. After we evaluated its contents together, my client cognitively determined that ice cream contained too many harmful ingredients. She threw away any remaining cartons she had in her freezer and ventured out to control her environment so it wasn't in the house. Life was organized in a way she didn't have to see or come in contact with any ice cream.

However, one day my client was at a party, and the forbidden treat appeared. The memory of the pleasurable but banned ice cream was still there. Trying to force a permanent prohibition of ice cream during massive job stress actually worked her brain into a frenzy while thinking about it. Since there was nothing as good in life as ice cream to her at the time, the memory escalated, and my client began compulsively seeking and consuming ice cream again, like an addict. Just like drugs can hijack the brain after habitual use, my client found that during a time of stress, ice cream had the same impact.

Before you decide to give up a food or beverage, work on maintaining a comfortable threshold of stress to allow your brain to focus. Or at a minimum, don't try to take on doing a major overhaul of your eating during major life events like during a move or while preparing for a wedding, going through a divorce, experiencing the death of a loved one, going through job loss or anticipating the birth of a child. I've worked with many people who made the mistake of trying to remodel their eating during a major transition in their lives. It didn't work. Before you take away foods or beverages during a time of chronic stress, first try some of the stress management techniques listed below.

Stress Management Techniques

Take Belly Breaths: When you have the urge to eat, first calm your mind and body by slowing down your breathing. Belly breathing stimulates your vagus nerve, which activates your relaxation response. This can be accomplished by these steps:

Step 1. Breathe through your nose, letting your belly fill with air. (Try saying in your mind, *I breathe in peace*.)

Step 2. Let the breath out through your nose. (Imagine the stress leaving your body with every breath.)

Step 3. Place one hand on your belly, the other on your chest. When you breathe in, feel your belly rise. When you breathe out, feel your belly drop. Be certain that the hand on your belly moves more than the hand on your chest.

Step 4. Repeat three times or until you feel relaxed.

Laugh: Before you look for food for comfort, lighten up by talking to someone you can smile and laugh with or tune into a favorite comedy. When you experience a good belly laugh, you lower your stress hormones (like cortisol) and increase feel-good hormones (like endorphins).

Work Out: When foods tempt you, at a minimum do a workout first before you let yourself indulge. Working out helps you release positive neurotransmitters and hormones and gives your brain the same kind of pleasure as eating synthetic foods. To increase your physical activity, go for a walk, bolt up and down a flight of stairs, or take a fitness class. All forms of exercise including yoga and stretching can help you release feel-good chemicals that enable you to combat anxiety and tension.

Problem Solve: As soon as you recognize that overeating synthetic foods is a problem for you, start to solve the issue. Focus on how good the outcome could be. Expect the best as you focus on possible solutions. Turn the pain of the problem into productive action. Get the courage to ask for help.

Practice Mindfulness and Meditation: Mindfulness is your ability to pay attention to what you are eating at the current moment. Meditation is an umbrella term encompassing mindfulness. When you meditate, your brain changes in positive ways. Both mindfulness and meditation enable you to control your reactions and perceptions of stressors and help you build new tools to deal with stress. For more on mindfulness and meditation, read on to the next chapter—Chapter 21.

After you set the stage at the right time, you'll have a greater ability to make a change. Some of my clients have stepped back away slowly and surely from synthetic foods, while others made an abrupt decision and never looked back. For whatever foods or beverages you think you can't live without, realize you are moving in the direction to one day be able to take it or leave it. Once the spell of needing a synthetic food, like my client did with ice cream, is broken, you can let go and choose real food from nature. You can begin the journey back to where your body belongs.

Chapter 21

Train Summary, Recommendations, and Action Steps

Step 3: Train

Train Your Brain to Form New Nerve Connections with Real Nature's Foods and Beverages

Training your brain to like nature's foods involves working on five areas mentioned in Chapters 15–20:

1. Override prior memories.
2. Establish new habits.
3. Train your taste buds and adjust your palate for new flavors.
4. Feed your gut to give your brain nourishment.
5. Undo stress to allow your brain to think properly.

My "Train" Experience

For years my normal lunch routine was to eat at a fast-food restaurant and grab a candy bar and soda at a convenience store afterward. My internal bell rang around lunchtime, and I began salivating for burritos, tacos, burgers, and milkshakes—all flavors of my favorites from places I had frequented.

After trying to eat better for a while, I found that I constantly went back to my old lunch routine. I rationalized, "It's not a big deal. My body can handle anything for one meal!" However, the problem wasn't that my body couldn't physically handle the extra load of protein, fat, saturated fat, trans fat, and sodium from time to time. The problem was that every time I consumed those foods and beverages, I prompted my brain to repetitively find and ingest them again. I was conditioning my gut and brain to like and want them more. With time and practice, habitual eating of synthetic foods became automatic, and when I tried to change the way I ate, my brain wanted to go back to what it knew. When my eating was automatic, I was free to focus away from what I was eating and pay attention to other things like the people around me or something I was reading. The synthetic foods went unconsciously into my mouth.

These seemingly innocent choices, repeated over and over again, were now fixed as a reward in my brain. Fast food, a candy bar and a soda didn't provide the nourishment my billions of body cells desperately needed. Insight and knowledge of the lack of nourishment I was receiving helped me identify that I was stuck in a habit loop (prompt, eat/drink, reward, repeat) of eating synthetic foods, and if I wanted to change, I needed to put some effort into training my brain to stop the loop.

After I decided to eat more of nature's foods, I made an effort to increase the amount of plant-based foods I was eating. I started packing my lunch more and eating out less, and over time at lunch hour, I surprisingly found that I was looking forward to eating my pre-made lunches. I confess that I didn't love vegetables at first, but slowly, after making changes in my eating, I noticed that my energy and moods were improving. Looking back, I realize that the pleasure of eating healthily, especially vegetables, initially happened more in my body than in my mind. I was thrilled with the increased stamina and mental clarity I was gaining. Also, once I ate specific vegetables over and over again, I began to enjoy their taste and form new memories. With the underlying belief that vegetables were an excellent choice for my cells and body, I began to understand more the reasons I was consuming them. My memories of the vegetables became more powerful because I put importance on the choice of consuming them. Little did I know that those meaningful memories are now the foundation for my desire to eat from nature today.

I specifically remember the day when I became aware of my shift in food preferences. After eating the lunch I had packed, I went to the local convenience store to grab a snack. Instead of going for my usual candy bar and soda, I walked around the store, looking for something else. I wanted something healthy but didn't find anything. After circling the store many times, I walked out empty handed. I remember standing outside the convenience store in a state of bewilderment, thinking, *What just happened?* I surprised myself that I didn't grab my usual snack. My internal bell wasn't ringing for a candy bar and soda, and I realized I was breaking free from the habit of eating synthetic foods.

Train Recommendations

Your brain doesn't behave like a computer that has a fixed algorithm of eating. It *can* be reprogrammed. Remember there is a process to change. Don't give up if and when you find yourself back in an unconscious eating or drinking episode with synthetic foods. Realize that it happens, and it's okay.

Because you are unique and have different sensory interactions, your journey along a better path will be exclusively your own. You are an individual whose life experiences speak to you alone. Try not to compare yourself to anyone else as you embark on your journey. The older you are, the more time you have had to routinely practice a certain way of eating and the more time it will take to modify your eating behaviors. Be patient with yourself during your change process. According to research, most adults need about 66 days [51] to practice new behaviors for them to be established as automatic and permanent. After practicing and practicing new habits, it still takes time for the nerves in your brain to rewire. I've discovered in my clients that a permanent shift to wanting nature's foods usually takes anywhere from one to two years or longer.

When you are ready to train your thoughts to routinely desire nature's foods, here are some tips:

- *Scrutinize why you feel the need to eat a certain food or drink a desired beverage.* If you find yourself eating or drinking a synthetic food or beverage, investigate and be hyperaware of why you're consuming the soda, cake, ice cream, chips, corn dog, cookies, and so forth. As long as your cognition is intact and not overridden by stress, you can make an educated judgment call. Knowing the why behind your food and beverage choices gives you the ability to discern whether you still want to continue the same behavior.
- *Utilize your natural necessity to eat an assortment of foods.* Repeated flavors from both synthetic *and* nature's food time and time again get uninteresting, resulting in "taste fatigue." That's why when you repeatedly eat the same foods, you eventually begin to forage for something new. Optimal health depends on your body receiving a variety of nutrients, so when this natural tendency to branch out to unique flavors occurs, use it to your advantage to seek nature's foods.
- *Eat three bites of produce first.* When you start craving something sweet or salty, eat three bites of a fruit or vegetable first (an apple or cucumber works well), and then see if you still really need or want that sugary or salty food. If, after you consume the fruit or vegetable, you end up eating the sweet or salty snack anyway (which many do), realize that by going for the produce first, you are in the training process of creating new habits and developing new memories that will override deep-rooted patterns of automatically choosing sweet or salty foods.
- *Nourish your brain.* When you begin to nourish your brain with foods that contain antioxidants, your brain uses these powerful chemicals to generate new nerve connections. A nourished brain helps you prevent diseases and promotes healthier aging. What's more, animal research studies show that the nutrients in nature's foods, especially flavanol-rich foods like legumes, apples, citrus fruits, berries, tomatoes, romaine lettuce, green tea, and 72 percent or more dark chocolate, positively boost the brain by increasing the function of the hippocampus, the memory and learning center of the brain. [142] Good foods help you remember

and think. *Healthier brains come from eating nature's foods, and a healthier brain helps you be your best self.* Think of your amazing potential. Nature's foods will help you get there.

- *Use dopamine.* As discussed earlier, dopamine is the pleasure and teaching neurotransmitter and is activated when you eat foods high in sugar, fat, and salt, but it is also secreted during physical activity. Since nobody wants a life absent of pleasure, *the next time a temptation to consume a synthetic food is strong, do something active instead, like going for a walk outdoors. The brain receives similar pleasurable results.*

- *Practice mindfulness and meditation.* When you meditate, your brain changes in positive ways. Meditation and mindfulness practices are associated with neuroplastic (new neural connection) changes in distinct areas of your brain, and these changes can be made throughout your life. [138] Meditating successfully has nothing to do with how still your mind is. In reality, during meditation your mind is busy. Multiple areas of your brain are activated like a switchboard, lighting up and trying to connect and work in tandem. Over time multiple meditation events strengthen these connections and positively rewire your brain.

    One of the most pleasing effects of meditation can be seen by how much more adaptable you are in your life. Most of my clients admit that meditation helps them handle the stressors of the day better. Also, meditation increases your capacity for open and receptive attention to present-moment eating experiences. [147] This means you become better at paying attention to what's going on at any given moment, which translates into being attentive to your food choices. Here is an additional list of benefits that come from meditation.

    - It helps you focus your attention and anticipate rewards.
    - It regulates your blood pressure and heart rate.
    - It helps you to make good decisions.
    - It can enhance your ethics and morals.
    - It assists you in seeing yourself positively.
    - It cultivates your creativity, intuition, and compassion.

- It controls your impulses and emotions.
- It has been associated with a reduction in depression and anxiety and an increase in happiness, relaxation, and emotional balance. [64]

Both mindfulness and meditation are responsible for helping you create a heightened awareness of yourself and your actions toward foods and beverages. When it comes to eating, being mindful helps you to pay attention to what's going in your mouth. Eating mindfully draws attention to the foods you consume while you're eating them. During your shift to eat more from nature, increased awareness can give you the strength to stay the course.

Action Steps for Step 3: Train

1. Practice

Learning to seek real foods from nature takes practice and isn't an overnight process. There are new nerve signals that need training. When healthy foods are introduced to your palate for the first time, you may reject them. If so, don't give up. Remember, in my experience, it can take a minimum of six attempts (on average) of trying a vegetable or a new food before your brain will begin to accept it. For long-term success, it's best to gradually swap in nature's foods rather than to try to exchange everything at once. Slowly but surely you will begin to desire nature's flavors more.

2. Visualize Your Future Self Enjoying Real Foods from Nature

Once you decide to consume nature's foods, see yourself mentally as if you're already there. If you can imagine yourself eating and drinking real foods from nature, you can achieve that state of being. Change your thoughts by starting with "I am," then end with words that define you as if you are already living in your identified desired state of being. For example, say, "I am enjoying a healthy body by eating a wide variety of produce" or "I'm lean, healthy, energetic, and fit." Hold on to the ideal image of yourself as if you are already there. Write down your phrase and look at it often. Make it part of your meditation practice. Let the catchphrase you develop become your mantra, a statement you repeat over and over again to aid concentration. It's amazing how this works. I've seen people shed weight that began by visualizing themselves in a smaller size. I've also seen those who were in pain for years literally become pain free after they practiced both saying to themselves, "I'm pain free" and mentally seeing themselves living without pain.

When you write down and begin to focus on your directional phrase, you program your subconscious mind to move in that direction. This helps your brain establish ownership of the new state of being. If you want to be leaner and healthier with more energy, design mental images of yourself living a lean, healthy, and energetic life. Or if you want to take up running, put in your mind an image of yourself finishing your first 5K race with a smile on your face. Visualize and verbalize what you want your life, health, and appearance to be. You will be able to get to that ideal self faster by first seeing yourself already there.

Keep in mind that programming your subconscious will take repetition and imagery. If you simply say or imagine something once, you will forget it, guaranteed. Rather, repeat your phrase and visualize the image of your healthiest self multiple times a day. Some of my clients set a timer and repeat their phrases every time the timer rings—morning, evening, and night. Others repeat it every time they eat a meal or snack.

Use the space below to write your catchphrase (or mantra).

    Fill in the blank.
    At my best self,

I am_____.

Create the image of the healthiest version of you. Draw or explain it below.

Repeat your "I am" phrase and visualize the image of your best self every hour or every time you eat for the first week and then regularly from then on. When you wake up, have your phrase in your mind. When you eat lunch, repeat and visualize it. When you go to bed, repeat and visualize it. Establish a routine of repeating your phrase and seeing yourself in your desired state.

3. **Manage Stress through Meditation**

Stress hormones can interrupt your ability to rewire your brain. Thoughts like *Should I consume this or not?* are not activated during stress. To cope with life's stressors, engage in some effective stress-reduction practices like mindfulness or meditation or practice stress-management techniques like deep breathing, laughing, and/or working out.

Beginning a Meditation Practice

If you have a difficult time settling down during the day, try meditating either before you go to bed or make it the first thing you do when you get up. If you're new to meditation, start small. Begin by trying it for thirty seconds or a short amount of time and extend the time as the practice feels more restful.

This simple "I am" meditation can get you started. It helps your mind focus on your desired state and your future ideal self.

> ### "I Am" Meditation
>
> Lie down or sit in a chair with your feet grounded on the floor. Close your eyes, progressively relax all the muscles in your body, and focus on finishing the phrase: *At my best self, I am _____*. Sync your phrase or mantra with your breathing. See yourself as if you are already living the life you desire. When your thoughts turn to other things (and they will), focus your mind back on your phrase or pay attention to the shift in your breath as it goes from inhalation to exhalation, and vice versa. After thirty seconds or a comfortable amount of time, come back slowly as you count backward from five to one. Wiggle your fingers and toes, shrug your shoulders, and then open your eyes.

After you feel comfortable with the "I am" style of meditation, progress toward "Nature'sMindfulness Meditation" found in Chapter 28.

My Meditation Experience

Personally, since I've been meditating, I've noticed how calm I am in situations that previously caused me to get upset. Meditation has allowed me to think through my reactions before I blow. I can honestly say I have more joy in my life. I feel that I have the ability to identify and regulate my emotions better now that I meditate. I also attribute my capacity to eat well and take care of my body as two healthy outcomes of meditation. After years of practice, I feel that I'm instinctively mindful about the quantity and quality of food I put in my body and how full I feel after a meal. Meditation has changed my eating and life for the better.

The next section gives a holistic approach to how to eat real food and love it. After training your mind and body to seek nature's food, your next step is to take care of other areas of your life. Real foods from nature give you the energy to support a healthy lifestyle. Most people who are typically well nourished want to make overall health changes and simultaneously work on the other two pillars of health—exercise and meditation. These three pillars together—eating, exercise, and mindfulness—are the keys to refining your health completely. All three pillars are covered in "Step 4: Unite."

STEP 4

U

Unite clean eating with exercise and meditation to form a healthy, natural lifestyle.

Chapter 22

Unite Your Foods to Work for You

*When you welcome the right food into your body,
your muscles and mind celebrate.*

Step 4: Unite

Eating

A. Develop a consistent, healthy eating routine. When you regularly practice new behaviors of eating, you create healthy long-term habits. Over time your body and mind begin to crave this new way.

Nature's Eating Tips

- Consume foods and beverages throughout the day. Use one or both of these methods for spacing foods:
  1. Eat your breakfast within two hours of waking and eat every four to five hours thereafter.
  2. End your eating eight to twelve hours after you begin.
- Use Nature's Food Selection Guide to plan your meals and consume the right balance of foods. You can also follow an

expanded meal plan, complete with a specific four-week meal plan and recipes, available at Thenatureshift.com.

Exercising

B. Engage in physical activity daily. Move your muscles regularly to build your body and help your brain reduce cravings for synthetic foods while increasing cravings for nature's foods. See exercise suggestions in Chapter 27.

Meditating

C. Cultivate a regular meditation routine. If you're new to meditation, begin with the "I am" meditation in Chapter 21, Progress to "Nature's Meditation" in Chapter 28.

Elizabeth's "Unite" Journey toward Eating Nature's Foods

Initially, Elizabeth confessed that eating real food was boring and that she felt deprived at events when she chose not to eat her usual favorites. However, this also made her realize how much she relied on food and beverages to perk up her mood and feel part of her social network. But as she continued eating nature's foods, she discovered that the natural sweetness of fruit, when picked at peak ripeness, tasted just as good to her as a cookie. The kick she used to get from synthetic foods she now got from nature's foods. She ate healthily, didn't feel deprived, and realized that her friends and family members were starting to notice a difference in her.

As Elizabeth began to meditate daily, she discovered that, with her added energy and happier moods, she found pleasure in other activities not involving food. Elizabeth joined a pickleball team, which gave her a new social and physical outlet she enjoyed. She also took plant-based cooking classes and got involved in prepping breakfasts and lunches with a friend. Both of these activities gave her palate exciting new flavors, and she liked that nature's foods were convenient and stimulating.

Food Confliction: Eating Is Confusing

Let's talk about the trends and opinions of food today. If you live in the United States, you are blessed to be in a time and place of food and beverage abundance. Yet Americans are bombarded with conflicting information about diets, supplements, brands, and which magic concoctions can prevent diseases. Over the last few decades, I've seen foods go on and off the "bad" and "good" lists as if they were criminals for a time, set free, then locked away again. They are judged in society by variables like staunch beliefs of how the food will affect health outcomes, how a said food will help you lose or gain weight, and/or which doctor or celebrity endorsed what food or diet. Meat, carbs, milk, vegetable oils, soy, eggs, gluten, low fat, Atkins, South Beach, Blood Type, Zone, Fen-Phen, Keto, and Paleo all come to mind as some food and diet controversies I've seen throughout the years. With so much information available, it's difficult to choose the correct course of action if you are seeking to be fit and healthy.

To maneuver through the food confusion, you can follow Nature's Food Selection Guide in Chapter 26. As you are eating foods from nature, focus on your individuality and try to understand what your body needs. Pay attention to your unique physique and try not to compare yourself to anyone else. One thing is clear: your DNA and body are one of a kind. There is no one exactly like you. With time and practice, you will understand your body and learn what foods build you up and what foods act like sledgehammers in your system. When you have tapped into eating real food regularly, your body will tell you what it likes and what it doesn't. You'll be able to rely on your internal wisdom to make choices that best suit you. Throughout my years of diet counseling, I have had to coach people to embrace their physiology and eat according to their own needs. The foods that work for my clients are sometimes counterintuitive to the latest fad of the day, but when they see results, they become believers.

When to Eat

Timing Makes All the Difference

Before you begin figuring out what to eat, pay attention to *when* you eat. Those who consume breakfast within two hours of waking and eat every four to five hours thereafter can manage their blood sugars and prevent intense cravings for synthetic foods, especially sweet ones. The combination of foods on Nature's Food Selection Guide in Chapter 26, is designed to help you feel full after you eat them, thus providing you with a natural spacing between your meals and snacks. Eating food every four to five hours throughout the day or a snack three hours after a meal has been the ideal spacing for me and most of my clients.

The timing of eating has become a hot topic with the trend of intermittent fasting. The word *intermittent* means occurring at irregular intervals. Two of the major techniques for intermittent fasting include (1) alternate-day fasting, in which you fast one to four days a week or eat five days and fast for two; and (2) early-time-restricted feeding (eTRF), which recommends that you start your eating early in the day and consume your foods within a four- to ten-hour window. With this method, you end up fasting for 14-20 hours. The "early" in the eTRF recommendation is based on hormonal rhythms. Because hormones that regulate your metabolism, like cortisol, growth hormone, and insulin, are secreted in cadence with your circadian rhythm, this method theorizes that it's best to eat in the morning when these hormones peak, then taper off eating in the evening. [72] Studies show that if you are looking to lose weight, eTRF is the preferred method of the two fasting techniques to assist you in the process.

Again, eating your food every four to five hours throughout the day has been the most successful meal spacing I've seen in terms of health and weight. However, since everyone is different, Nature's Food Selection Guide can work into eTRF. You can shrink your allowable eating time to an eight- to ten-hour window, although personally I practice a 12 hour eating window and do just fine. A ten-hour fast would mean your first meal would begin at 8 a.m., and your last would end at 6 p.m. Trying to consume all the plants in Nature's Food Selection Guide in a four-hour eating window can be problematic and cause gas, bloating, and indigestion due to the intense fiber load you would need to eat in a short amount of time. Your body needs time to digest foods previously eaten.

Chapter 23

Unite Activity with Eating to Run Your Metabolism

In this chapter, I will attempt to share with you how your body uses and stores food energy. To illustrate calorie storage and calorie burn, I'm going to talk scientifically about how your body functions by using some medical terms. As you read through the sections on calories, I encourage you to keep in mind that not all calories are created equally. Nature's foods get metabolized and support the function of your body differently than synthetic foods. They have powerful antioxidant abilities to protect your cells, whereas the calories you eat from synthetic foods don't. It's the quality of the calories you eat that matters.

Energy from Food

Calorie Burn

Your body is made up of trillions of cells, and each cell needs an energy source for power. After the foods you eat are broken down, they create a compound called "adenosine triphosphate" (ATP). This is the fuel source that breaks apart and provides energy for your body to function. The location where ATP is stored and created into chemical energy inside your body cell is called your "mitochondria." These are tiny powerhouses that process and generate energy. On average there are from one thousand to twenty-five hundred mitochondria living inside each of your body's cells, [123] meaning that you have the potential of generating a significant amount of energy.

If you're trying to lose fat weight, build your muscle tissue to acquire more mitochondria and more ATP. Since muscles are the most active of all your organs and tissues in your body, as noted, muscle activity creates more mitochondria, which burns through calories like the roar of a fire blazing through a pile of tinder. With an increase of mitochondria, your body needs more calories to feed the demanding muscle tissue. Weightlifting and physical labor are ways to build your muscles to yield a higher mitochondrial density and higher calorie burn. As you age, unless you follow an active lifestyle, your muscles will decline, and the number of mitochondria you have in your muscles will concurrently decrease as well. [77] When you lose muscle, called "sarcopenia," out goes your mitochondria, which may leave you feeling fatigued.

On the contrary, calories stored in the form of fat burn slowly, like the prolonged burn of charcoal. This type of burn fosters a conserved, gradual release of energy. With the right balance of nature's foods, you receive the right type of calories to feed the demands of your active muscle tissue while also providing fuel to your slow-burn warehouse of stored calories—your fat cells.

Calorie Storage

Glycogen or Triglycerides

Let's take a look at the way calories are stored. Your body has two forms of calorie storage: glycogen (carbohydrate storage) and triglycerides (fat storage). Glycogen is basically long chains of glucose (blood sugar) molecules packed together. Your glycogen stores are for immediate use, like having cash on hand for instant purchases, whereas triglycerides are saved for energy needs when glycogen runs low or needs to be maintained, like pulling from your retirement savings plan. Triglycerides are stored in your fat cells located in your adipose tissue. Fat cells act like a bank. If you walked into any bank with extra money, the bank would gladly take it. The same with fat cells. They happily accept and accommodate additional calories that might be needed for later use. Let us explore each storage system a little further.

Glycogen: Carbohydrate Storage

The majority of your glycogen is stored in your muscles and liver, and a small amount of glycogen circulates throughout your bloodstream. On average your muscles store 400 grams of glycogen to give them power when needed. Your liver stores about 100 grams of glycogen, mostly to fuel your brain, and an additional 25 grams circulate throughout your bloodstream. [11] If you add up the glycogen grams and convert them to calories, you will find that your body has roughly 2,000 calories worth of rapidly available fuel for instant needs. Therefore, when food isn't readily available, your body will have quick energy to use when necessary. Glycogen can be quickly broken down into glucose molecules to be used for immediate energy needs.

Triglycerides: Fat Storage

Triglycerides make up the other storage form of calories in your body. Your fat cells can pile up triglycerides when you eat more than your cells require and in a warehouse-like fashion will form a reservoir of calorie storage for long-term use. That way calories can be accessed for possible emergencies but in places where you probably don't want them like your hips, thighs, and belly. As a matter of fact, your fat cells are so accepting and inviting that they can expand to create room for extra calorie storage. Fat cells range in size starting at 20 µms and distend to 300 µm [144] in diameter (the term *µm* stands for micrometer, which is an incredibly small unit of measurement—about 0.000039 of an inch). And once all your thirty trillion or so fat cells are stretched to capacity, they will happily accommodate more storage by dividing and creating more room (or more fat cells) to increase their triglyceride depositories. Fortunately, for survival sake, but unfortunately for disease and body weight, once your fat cells are stretched to capacity, they will divide and store calories until fully stretched, then divide again, store calories until fully stretched, and continue on and on exponentially as long as excess calories are coming in. This fat adaptation is your body's way of protecting itself. Should days of famine arrive, your fat cells will pull from your inventory of calorie storage to keep you alive.

It's an interesting phenomenon that the more fat you have in your body, the more efficient you get at storing it. The higher the concentration of fat cells, the more efficient triglycerides get at slipping right into your fat cells. With excess fat on board, your brain thinks it's in survival mode and helps your body ramp up its packaging system. It wants you to keep extra calories hidden away for the long haul. An overabundance of calories reassures your brain that you will be able to stay alive in a famine (even though it's unlikely in industrialized countries). When more fat comes into the fat cells, there is a higher demand for storage.

To assist in the fat-storing process, your fat calls secrete higher levels of two important hormones—leptin and adiponectin. Like any business, your fat cells create a supply chain network with workers to meet the demand. Leptin is similar to the sales team of a business, wanting to find more calories, and adiponectin acts like the building maintenance crew, slowing down the overall exit of its inventory—the calorie supply. The job of leptin is to increase your appetite, and the function of adiponectin is to decelerate your metabolism. [28] When these two hormones take over the command centers of the fat cells, your appetite can be voracious and your metabolism sluggish. This condition leaves you primed to forage for high-calorie synthetic foods and beverages ... and devour them.

Over the years I've worked with many clients stuck in this hormonal surge. Even though they intended to change their eating so they could lose weight or improve their health, they found themselves overindulging in synthetic foods and wondering why. It was because their hormones were doing their job to keep the warehouses of fat stores full. This situation, combined with the ability to afford large amounts of synthetic foods, leads to the obesity epidemic we see today. If you find yourself in this category, realize that hormonal changes take time to reset. Be patient on your road to change. Over time your hormones will readjust.

Muscle Movement

Using the analogy that leptin acts like the sales team trying to get more inventory (calories) to pack the warehouses (fat cells), and your adiponectin is the building maintenance crew regulating how much inventory can leave, let's add other members to the team—myokines. Myokines are hormones muscles secrete that act like the foremen of the team. (More on myokines in Chapter 27.) They can be brought in to move the inventory out of the warehouses to other locations. In contrast to fat storage, if you continually move your muscles, you get an accelerated calorie burn, and your body gets the message that muscle mass, not fat, is in greater need of your calories.

For example, when you work your muscles during resistance, like doing push-ups, you activate your muscles. If the push-ups keep going, your muscles quickly burn through their quick-energy glycogen stores to meet the demand of the working muscles and then look around your body for additional calories to keep the fires burning. This is when your warehouse of fat is called on to meet the energy needs of the demanding muscle. Triglycerides are then broken down to feed your active muscles. Therefore, the trick to avoiding unnecessary fat storage is to build and strengthen your muscles through movement, especially through resistance training and high-intensity interval training (HIIT). These two methods of training help your metabolism deliver calories to your muscles instead of your fat cells, and you become more efficient at breaking down fat to help feed your muscles. *Bottom line: if you want your muscles to use your calories, move them; otherwise excess calories will get stored as fat.*

Scale Weight

After three decades of working in the medical field, I am baffled that the unit of measurement still collected and recorded to reflect a patient's physical progress is his or her scale weight. The weight on a scale gives only a snapshot of what is going on in the body. Extra weight on a scale could mean you are retaining fluids or gaining muscle mass; or it could simply mean your bowels are full. I've worked with so many people over the years who base their happiness on what the scale says. If their weight is up, they are annoyed, frustrated, depressed, and sometimes panicked. If their weight is down, they analyze what they did. They want to repeat whatever actions they did to lose weight, even if their actions aren't healthy.

It's difficult to convince my patients who are trying to lose fat weight that if their clothes are loose, they are losing fat. For many, it's been drilled into their minds that a number on a scale means they are doing right or wrong behaviors. I recommend that if you're trying to lose weight, when you shift to nature's foods, assess your progress by getting a tape measure and recording four measurements on yourself: your chest, waist, hips, and thighs. Routinely check your measurements instead of your scale weight. If you're losing inches, you are losing fat. As your inches go down, celebrate the fact that you're losing the right kind of weight—fat weight. You can record your measurements on the TNS food symptoms record form found on Thenatureshift.com website.

Breathe the Fat Out

Speaking of fat loss, I have seen a lot of it in my clients over the years. A person looks very different at 150 pounds if his or her starting weight was 225. When the warehouses of calories in the form of triglycerides in your fat cells are depleted, there is a visual difference. Clusters of fat cells are directly beneath the skin; when these cells deplete, the entire person shrinks. If you have ever wondered how fat exits your body when someone loses weight, biochemists have discovered the answer. Contrary to the popular belief that your fat cells dissipate into energy, it's now understood that fat mainly leaves the body through your breath. To explain this, I will use a little chemistry.

When you put a triglyceride molecule under a microscope, you will see that it is made up of carbon, hydrogen, and oxygen. During weight loss (or fat loss), your fat cells are broken down for energy, and the final end products are carbon dioxide (CO_2) and water (H_2O). [101] Your body uses the basic ingredients of stored carbon and oxygen from your fat cells to make CO_2 and concurrently uses hydrogen and oxygen to make H_2O. To be specific, 84 percent of the breakdown of your fat turns into carbon dioxide, and 16 percent turns into water. Interestingly, when your muscles are actively exercising and you are breathing hard, carbon dioxide is exhaled through your lungs. Water, the other end product, leaves your body through urination, bowel movements, sweat, and so forth. You know you're getting a good workout when you're breathing hard but realize that the actual act of that deep, fast breathing is also the exit route after your fat is broken down. [101]

Metabolic Rate

When a fire is lit, it needs fuel to keep burning. Similarly, maintaining human cell function requires calories as the fuel source to keep them functioning. Cells need a regular supply of energy to power basic body movements such as breathing, brain functioning, and blood circulation. The amount of fuel required to maintain these basic functions is referred to as your resting metabolic rate (RMR). Your RMR accounts for up to 70 percent of your total metabolism. The remaining 30 percent of your metabolism is needed for digestion, exercise, and non-exercise activity thermogenesis (NEAT), which includes everyday tasks like walking from the kitchen to the living room, getting dressed, cooking meals, and so forth. For all the body cells to receive enough fuel, a typical woman needs approximately 1,200-1,500 calories a day, and a typical man needs approximately 1,500-1,800 calories per day. [84] For extra movement, an additional three hundred to fifteen hundred calories are needed, depending on the movement's intensity and duration. The number of extra calories required for each person depends on multiple factors like age, weight, fitness level, sex, height, the amount and type of exercise, and so forth. For example, a person who weighs 150 pounds could burn anywhere from 70 to 170 calories per hour at rest, depending on the factors listed above. *Basically, the taller, younger, and more muscular you are, the more calories you need.*

Mifflin-St Jeor Equation

A mathematical way to see how many calories your body needs is to calculate your basal metabolic rate (BMR), the rate your body burns calories while at rest, using the Mifflin-St Jeor equation. This equation uses your gender, weight, height, and age to calculate your basal metabolic rate (BMR), multiplied by a factor with a value between 1.2 and 1.9, depending on your activity level. If you choose to use this equation, please keep in mind that not all body functions are well understood, so calculating total daily caloric needs from BMR estimates is just that, an estimate.

If you don't like math equations, you can also find online calculators to find your BMR. Here's one you can try:

https://www.calculator.net/bmr-calculator.html.

Phase 1: Determine the number of calories you need to run your BMR.

Male	BMR = (10 × weight in kg)* + (6.25 × height in cm)** - (5 × age in years) + 5
Female	BMR = (10 × weight in kg)* + (6.25 × height in cm)** - (5 × age in years) - 161

*(weight in kg = weight in pounds divided by 2.2)
** (height in cm = height in inches x 2.54)

Using this equation, a 150-pound (68 kg) woman measuring five feet and five inches (sixty-five inches or 165 cm) who is fifty years old would need 1,302 calories a day to run her BMR.

Phase 2: Multiply by a factor with a value between 1.2 and 1.9.

Once your BMR calorie needs are established, multiply the result by a physical activity level (PAL) to determine your total energy expenditure (TEE) or the total number of calories you need per day. The daily caloric need is your BMR value found by the Mifflin-St Jeor equation multiplied by a factor with a value between 1.2 and 1.9, depending on your activity level.

Physical Activity Level Calculation

Activity Level	Activity Factor
Sedentary Little to no exercise	1.2
Lightly Active Two hours of walking around during a day	1.375
Moderately Active Three hours of walking around during a day or moderate exercise three to five days per week	1.55
Very Active Four hours of walking around during a day or hard exercise six to seven days per week	1.725
Extremely Active Five hours of walking around during a day including hard daily exercise	1.9

Adjusting for PAL, a very active 150-pound (68 kg) woman who is five foot and five inches (sixty-five inches or 165 cm) tall and is fifty years old needs 1,302 calories a day for her BMR according to the Mifflin-St Jeor equation. She will need 2,246 calories a day (1,302 x 1.725) to meet her TEE.

Factors That Influence Your Caloric Needs

- Muscle mass: The more muscle mass, the higher your BMR.
- Height: The taller you are, the greater the overall mass, and the higher your BMR.
- Genetics: Hereditary traits passed down from ancestors influence your BMR.
- Weather: Extreme cold or hot environments raise your BMR.
- Diet: Small, routinely dispersed meals increase your BMR.

- Pregnancy: Ensuring the livelihood of a separate fetus internally increases your BMR.
- Hormonal changes: Hormones can increase or decrease your BMR.

Another way to help you determine how many calories are most accurate for your particular body is record keeping as discussed in "Step 1: Notice." Keep track of the calories you both consume and expend and make needed adjustments over time. You can record your calories on the TNS food and symptoms record form found at Thenatureshift.com website.

Variables to Metabolism and Calories Needed

Discover how many calories you need a day. If you eat too many, as noted earlier, the excess gets stored as fat. On the other hand, consuming too few calories will result in muscle wasting and low energy. If you routinely consume an adequate number of calories and aren't able to see positive bodily changes, you may have an underlying hormonal (like low testosterone) or metabolic (like low-functioning thyroid) issue interfering with your ability to improve. This requires a visit to your physician.

Chapter 24

Unite Water with the Right Macros

What to Drink and Eat

Now that we have explored how our bodies use calories, let's take a more in-depth look at what to drink and eat.

Water, Water, Water: Nine to Thirteen Cups

Water is the most critical nutrient you can ingest. The Institute of Medicine has determined that sedentary men require three liters or thirteen cups of water per day, and sedentary women require two and two-tenths (2.2) liters or nine cups per day. [130] Of course, like the correct food intake, water needs are individualized. Keep in mind, however, that if you are engaged in physical activity or are exposed to higher temperatures, you will require even more water to maintain optimum hydration. Water aids in lubricating your joints, boosting your skin health, flushing out body wastes, and regulating your body's temperature. Drinking carbonated beverages, energy shots, sports drinks, juices, or alcoholic beverages cannot replace the need for water. Acids, sugar, high-intensity sweeteners, and alcohol contain toxins your body has to battle. Just drink clean, filtered water free of chemicals and additives. To add flavor to your water, try infusing it with fruits, vegetables, and/or herbs. Here are some of my favorite combinations:

Infused Water Combinations

Cucumber + lime + mint
Strawberry + lemon + basil
Cucumber + watermelon + lime
Blueberry + lemon + basil
Strawberry + basil + vanilla bean
Pineapple + cucumber + mint
Green apple + raspberries + rosemary
Orange + lemon + lime
Lemon + raspberries + mint
Blueberry + lemon + mint
Blackberry + cherries + lime
Lemon + cucumber + mint
Pineapple + orange + grated ginger
Citrus + cilantro
Kiwi + blackberry
Fennel + pear
Melon + basil
Lemon + lavender
Lime + ginger slices
Watermelon + mint

Directions: Mix all ingredients with a long spoon inside a pitcher, infusion water dispenser, or infusion water bottle. The flavors get stronger the longer the time they have to infuse. For variety, try seltzer or sparkling mineral water.

Regarding hydration, keep in mind that real foods from nature like fruits and vegetables will help increase your fluid intake even more. Nature's foods have a larger water content than dry foods and give a water source to your body when you eat them.

In the next section, we'll talk about each macronutrient: carbohydrates, protein, and fats. In nutrition vernacular, we typically call carbs, protein, and fats "macros." Again, I intend to help explain why the calories and macros from nature's foods are superior to those from synthetic foods.

Carbohydrate Fuel

With the popularity of low-carb approaches like the Keto and the Paleo diets, carbohydrates have been maligned as a nutrient to avoid. However, if you are worried about your weight, eat the largest portion of complex carbs (fiber-rich foods) at your first meal, a small amount at your second meal and then avoid them or just have three small bites at your third meal. Carbohydrates provide your cells with energy, and they will power your body and assist you. They do this by breaking down starch molecules into glucose quicker than proteins or fats. From simple breathing to running at full speed, your body needs easy access to glucose that can be quickly turned into energy. And the greatest consumer of glucose in your body is your brain.

Your brain requires a continuous dose of glucose to run properly. As we learned in Chapter 16, even though your brain weighs only about three pounds, it requires 20 percent of all the glucose-derived calories you eat. This means that if you eat 2,100 calories a day, 420 of those calories (120 g of glucose) will go directly to your brain. [44] The reason your brain requires a steady supply of glucose is that it needs to power the billions of brain neurons actively working to keep you alive and functioning at full capacity. If carbohydrates aren't available, you generate ketone bodies in your liver, which are partly used to replace glucose as a fuel source. [11] The secretion of ketones is a hallmark of the word *ketosis*. Studies show that your brain will use ketone bodies instead of glucose when ketones are present. Ketone bodies meet your brain's energy needs but are best used in a short-term situation. [32]

The Dietary Reference Intakes by the Food and Nutrition Board, Institute of Medicine, recommends that adults consume 45 to 65 percent of their calories from carbohydrates, 10 to 35 grams from protein, and 20 to 35 percent from fat. [38] Since the highest percentage of your calorie needs comes from carbohydrates, they are ubiquitous in both foods from nature and synthetic foods.

How Carbohydrates Are Converted into Energy

After you eat carbohydrates, enzymes break them down in your digestive tract. Your digestive tract is an amazing organ. Here's the process carbohydrates go through to make energy for your body: A carbohydrate-rich food is initially broken down into smaller particles when an enzyme, called "salivary amylase," is secreted in your mouth during chewing. As carbohydrates enter your stomach, additional enzymes break them down farther into even smaller pieces. From the stomach, the broken-down particles enter your small intestines, where they get converted into glucose and are carried through the bloodstream to your cells. When glucose nears the front door of each cell, your pancreas secretes the hormone insulin, which acts as a key to open the door of the cell to allow glucose to enter. As discussed earlier, in the mitochondria of the cell, your cells use glucose to make the energy source adenosine triphosphate (ATP) to power your cells.

The reason why low-carbohydrate diets work so well for immediate weight loss is that with every gram of glycogen stored in your liver and muscles, your body stores three grams of water. [48] In other words, carbo*hydrates* hydrate your body. When access to carbohydrates is limited, your body is forced to use its glycogen stores for fuel, and out goes the water stored with it. Around two kilograms (4.4 pounds) of water will be excreted in the first few days as your glycogen is depleted and instant weight loss happens on the scale from the water loss. If your only goal is for scale numbers to be lower, a low-carbohydrate regimen will do the trick.

Complex and Simple Carbohydrates

There are two types of carbohydrates—complex and simple. When I hear my clients talk about eating "too many carbs," they are referring to eating too many simple carbohydrates that come from the white flour and sugar in synthetic foods. I rarely hear my clients struggling from eating too many complex carbs from nature's foods. No one says his or her weight gain is because they binged on barley, lentils, split green peas, or butternut squash. That's because complex carbohydrates are full of fibers that cause dissension and a delayed emptying in your stomach after you eat them. Since they gradually leave your stomach on their way to your small intestines, they don't raise your blood sugar like the refined sugars found in synthetic foods do. The fibers from complex carbs quickly fill you up, giving you an automatic shut-off switch from overconsuming them. Complex carbohydrates in nature's foods also provide vitamins, minerals, antioxidants, and fiber that help your body digest, absorb, and metabolize what you eat. As discussed earlier, the fiber in nature's food also acts as a fertilizer to your microbiome, helping it build a bulletproof wall of healthy microbes to strengthen your immune system. [131]

Simple carbohydrates (sugars) are found in both nature's foods and synthetic foods. However, the simple sugars in nature's foods like fructose are surrounded by fiber and nutrients. In contrast, the sugars you ingest from synthetic foods are from processed sweeteners sourced from numerous amounts of sweeteners, chosen by food manufacturers. Ones that may be familiar to you are cane sugar, raw sugar, corn syrup, honey, and brown sugar. Others, not so commonly known, include dextrose, barley malt, ethyl maltol, dextrin, diastatic malt, maltodextrin, and rice syrup. Simple carbohydrates also include ultra-processed grains (like white flour) and are frequently combined with sugars to make synthetic foods like chips, cookies, crackers, pastries, doughnuts, most cereals, candy, packaged bars, sweetened drinks, fruit drinks, etc.

Let's look at how the body breaks down and absorbs carbohydrates.

A complex carbohydrate food, like steel-cut oats, are full of fiber which takes time to break down in the digestive tract. Simple carbohydrates like white bread, on the other hand, are highly refined and travel quickly through your digestive tract. There are major differences between complex carbohydrates and simple carbohydrates. Here are four:

1. Complex carbohydrates create a gentle rise in your blood sugar compared to a sharp rise from simple carbs.
2. Complex carbohydrates stay in the digestive tract longer, giving you a sense of satiety or fullness.
3. Complex carbohydrates provide health-promoting fiber.
4. The quality of nutrients is superior in complex carbohydrates.

Nature's foods consist of complex carbohydrates. When choosing which kind of carbohydrates to eat, choose complex.

Protein: A Matrix of Amino Acids

Protein is a macronutrient that has been given the green light. While dieters have scrutinized and restricted carbohydrates and fats over the years, protein has remained untouched. Even though protein is a critical nutrient, it doesn't need to be the largest part of what you eat. Once your body reaches its daily quota of protein, any excess will either follow the same path as carbohydrates—converted into glucose and get stored as glycogen or be converted into triglycerides that enter your adipose tissue in the form of fat. There is no storage site on your body for extra protein. And just because protein comes into your body, it doesn't mean your cells will be able to use the protein to build and repair your muscles. Your body can handle only a limited amount.

The recommended daily allowance (RDA) of protein for adults is 0.8 grams of protein per kilogram or 0.36 per pound of body weight, which amounts to 54.5 grams for a 150-pound (68 kg) person. Yet protein requirements vary between each individual, and studies have shown that people who are 65 and older have increased protein needs of 1.0 to 1.2 grams of protein per kilogram. For bodybuilders, the daily need for protein may be as high as 1.2 to 1.7 grams of protein per kilogram or 0.5 to 0.75 grams per pound. [94]

After you eat food that contains protein, whether it's a plant food like quinoa or an animal food like chicken, enzymes in your stomach called "pepsin" break down the proteins into amino acids. We know there are 22 amino acids that combine to form various proteins. Nine amino acids are considered essential, which means you need to consume them from nature because your body can't make them. The nine essential amino acids are phenylalanine, valine, tryptophan, threonine, isoleucine, leucine, lysine, histidine, and methionine. All nine are fully contained in animal products like eggs, meat, milk, yogurt, and cheeses; and in some plant foods like quinoa, buckwheat, and soybeans. If you see a plant food labeled as a "complete protein," it's to promote the fact that it uniquely has all nine essential amino acids. Other plant foods like whole grains, legumes, nuts, seeds, starchy vegetables, and vegetables are referred to as incomplete proteins because they have only a partial amount of essential amino acids.

Like Lego building blocks, amino acids are joined together in foods from nature. Once they are inside your digestive tract, enzymes split them apart so they can be used as precursors for your DNA [80] or used as building blocks to make proteins for molecules your body makes, such as neurotransmitters, muscle cells, hormones, antibodies, or collagen.

Real foods have an abundance of amino acids to help your immune system battle when pathogens infect your body. For example, the amino acid arginine helps generate the molecule nitric oxide (NO). [26] Nitric oxide recognizes patterns pathogens use to invade your cells and in response activates a defense network against the infectious organisms—kind of like a forensic scientist scoping out criminal patterns to stop their destructive behavior. Nitric oxide also dilates your blood vessels and keeps your arteries relaxed, allowing blood to flow freely throughout your body. You can get a good dose of arginine to make NO from nature's foods like nuts, whole grains, soybeans, pumpkin seeds, spinach, and spirulina—and especially in peanuts, which contain the highest amount of arginine of any plant food. [6]

If you choose, you can receive all your protein needs from plants.

Chart 4-A shows some plant foods that, when combined, provide all the essential amino acids you need.

Chart 4-A

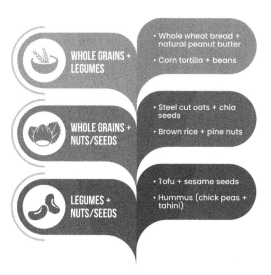

The combination of foods on chart 4-A contains essential amino acids and are packed full of vitamins and minerals. They are also free of chemicals and preservatives abundant in synthetic foods. Combining plant foods helps you maintain your body's sweet spot of protein needs. Keep in mind that you need a balance of plant foods to get the essential amino acids your body needs, but you don't need to eat them at the same time. As long as you eat whole grains, legumes, nuts, seeds, starchy vegetables, and vegetables within the same day, the nine essential amino acids stored in your liver will combine.

For your body to synthesize the protein you eat, space your protein intake throughout your day. For example, if you're a 150-pound person and you consume 0.8 to 1.7 grams of protein per kilogram or 0.36 per pound of body weight, your protein needs would be 54.5 to 115.6 grams a day. Use Table P to see how you can acquire the right amount of protein most people need per day. The times listed in the left column provide a good schedule for protein spacing. If you space your protein grams into four sessions, you would consume about 14 to 29 grams of protein per meal, depending on the number of calories you need. This schedule of protein spacing works well to build and repair muscle tissue, maintain even blood sugar levels, and avoid hunger pangs.

Table P: Spacing Protein Foods

Meal or Snack and Time Example	Plant Protein Ideas (14–29) Grams 1 ounce=7 grams	Non-Plant Protein Ideas (14–29 grams) 1 ounce=7 grams
Breakfast: 7–8 a.m.	4–6 oz scrambled tofu	Eggs: 2 whole
Lunch: 11 a.m.–noon	1/2–1 cup beans: black, pinto, garbanzo	2–4 oz tuna (water packed)
Snack: 2:30–3:30 p.m.	2–4 servings protein powder: hemp, pea, or soy (1 serving=7 g protein)	2–4 servings protein powder: egg or whey (1 serving=7 g protein)
Dinner: 5:30–6:30 p.m.	1/2–1 cup quinoa	2–4 oz poultry (skinless): chicken, Cornish hen, duck, pheasant, or turkey

Your Heart

When you increase high-quality protein foods and simultaneously decrease simple carbohydrates from your eating, your heart can function better. The national health statistics state that heart disease is the number one killer in the United States—a figure that has held the top position since 1921. [171] In essence, if you indulge in too many synthetic foods and beverages, the loss of the protective effects of antioxidants can contribute to the premature death of your most vital life force—your heart.

A condition called atherosclerosis is the main contributor to heart disease. Atherosclerosis is a condition where the arteries around your heart and throughout your body get plugged with a sticky substance called "plaque." Some people with good genetics can avoid the accumulation of plaque, but the majority of people who consume the standard American diet (a.k.a. SAD), which is full of synthetic foods, are at an increased risk of developing plaque build-up on their artery walls, which can eventually lead to a blockage of blood trying to get to and from the heart and other vital organs.

Doctors are reaching their limit as to what they can do to fight heart disease with medications, and because there is a growing epidemic of diabetes and obesity, progression toward suppressing these diseases has stalled. To shift the tide toward healing hearts, eating nature's foods instead of damaging arteries with synthetic foods is the way. With real food from nature, you can protect your cardiovascular health and reverse heart disease for the long haul. [46]

To prevent cardiovascular disease, the American Heart Association has created an online calculator you can use as a reference point to see whether you are at risk for disease. If you haven't already had a heart event, you can estimate your ten-year risk if you know your cholesterol numbers and blood pressure. Try this link if you want to check out your risk:
https://static.heart.org/riskcalc/app/index.html#!/baseline-risk

Fats: The Kind of Fat You Eat Matters

As previously mentioned, the wrong type of fats can build up in your bloodstream and lead to atherosclerosis. Over time, plaque can enlarge and cause a narrowing of your arteries. The final event is often a blood clot, which occludes whatever passageway it is in. If the blood vessels around your heart or brain become blocked, the eventual outcome is a heart attack or stroke. Researchers are finding that the type of fat you eat rather than the amount you eat contributes to an increased risk factor for atherosclerosis. [49] Some fat culprits abundant in synthetic foods are trans fats, rancid oils, too many foods high in saturated fats, and an elevated ratio of omega-6 to omega-3 fatty acids, which we will explore.

There are three types of naturally occurring fats—monounsaturated, polyunsaturated, and saturated—and one kind of manufactured fat called "trans fats."

Fats

- Monounsaturated
- Polyunsaturated—including omega-3 and omega-6 fatty acids
- Saturated
- Trans—manufactured

Trans Fats: The Man-Made Cloggers

Let's first look at trans fats and their chemical makeup. Trans fats are produced when hydrogen molecules are added to vegetable oils, causing them to become solid. After the hydrogenation process, vegetable oils are classified as either hydrogenated or partially hydrogenated. This transformation gives a product a longer shelf life. For example, when margarine is made, trans fats help it to be more firm, have greater plasticity, and possess a stabilized emulsion [37]—a bonus for a food company wanting to sell a spreadable margarine that can sit on a refrigerated shelf for months before it spoils. However, trans fats lead to excessive inflammation throughout your bloodstream. Inflammation is known to be the seed of chronic diseases like heart disease, stroke, and type 2 diabetes.

For years in the United States, food companies widely used trans fats to make their products; however, in March 2017, the FDA acknowledged that trans fats had a direct link to heart attacks and deaths. They set a compliance period of three years for food companies to remove all hydrogenated or partially hydrogenated oils from their foods. Trans fats no longer reside on the generally recognized as safe (GRAS) list and are therefore not allowed in the food supply.

The Ratio of Omega-6 Fatty Acids to Omega-3s

Food companies widely use lower-cost oils like corn oil, cottonseed oil, safflower oil, soybean oil, and/or sunflower oil to increase the shelf life of a food and improve the mouthfeel of their products. These oils are all high in an essential fat called omega-6 (linoleic) polyunsaturated fat. Consuming too many omega-6s has been linked to increased blood clots, inflammation, and weight gain. Studies show that people with heart disease consume a greater amount of omega-6 fats than those who don't have heart disease. [40]

Today we know that to prevent diseases, our bodies need a higher ratio of omega-3 (alpha-linolenic) fat to omega-6 fats. Both fats are *essential* because we must consume them for survival, but for good health we need more omega-3s. There is currently no set guideline for the ratio of omega-6 to omega-3 essential fatty acids (at the time of this writing), yet experts agree that a ratio of 1–2:1 omega-6/omega-3 is ideal. Before 1900, the ratio of omega-6 fatty acids to omega-3s was 1:1. Since then, with the significant addition of omega-6s to synthetic foods, the ratio has jumped to as high as 20:1 omega-6/omega-3s. With the higher ingestion of omega-6s, we have seen a parallel increase in obesity. [139] If you are curious to know whether you consume omega-6s, take a look at the ingredients in the packaged products you eat and see what kind of oil is in them.

By balancing your omega-6/omega-3 ratio to 1–2:1 and increasing your physical activity, you'll be making an important change to protect your health. Here are some suggestions that can help you increase your ratio of omega-3 fatty acids:

1. Decrease the amount of omega-6 fatty acids you consume like corn oil, cottonseed oil, safflower oil, soybean oil, and/or sunflower oil. By reducing your consumption of synthetic foods full of omega-6 oils, you'll begin to improve your omega-6/omega-3 ratio.
2. Consume more foods high in omega-3 fatty acids like chia seeds, flax seeds, hazelnuts, hazelnut oil, high monounsaturated sunflower oil, macadamia nuts, macadamia nut oil, olives, olive oil, walnuts, and walnut oil.
3. Increase your wild fish intake to two to three servings a week and decrease your overall meat intake.

Nature's Fats for Optimal Functioning

Even though fats can do damage in the blood stream, they are needed by the human body for survival. Eating nature's foods that contain fat is *essential*. However, you only need a small dose of them. For an adult who needs 1,500 calories a day, to receive the amount of essential fat needed, he or she needs to eat only 21 calories worth of an essential dietary fat source like nuts, seeds, avocado, or wild fish. This is the equivalent of two walnut halves, one and a half teaspoons of flaxseeds, half an ounce of avocado, or two tablespoons of wild fish.

The following table shows what foods are good sources of each fat. Each food you see listed actually contains a blend of monounsaturated, polyunsaturated, and saturated fats. They are placed in a specific category, depending on which type of fat is highest.

Fats	Foods
Monounsaturated	Avocado, avocado oil, canola oil *(high oleic), hempseeds, macadamia nuts, olive oil, olives (black, green kalamata)
Polyunsaturated	Almonds, almond oil, Brazil nuts, cashews, grape-seed oil, nut and seed butters, peanuts, pecan (halves), pine nuts, rice bran oil, seeds (sunflower, pumpkin, sesame), sesame oil, soy nuts
o High in Omega-3	Chia seeds, flaxseed (ground), flaxseed oil, hazelnuts, walnut (halves), walnut oil, wild-caught fish
o High in Omega-6	Corn oil, cottonseed oil, mayonnaise (unsweetened), safflower oil (high oleic), soybean oil, sunflower oil (high oleic)
Saturated	Butter (grass fed), coconut dried, coconut milk, coconut oil, ghee (clarified butter), palm kernel, palm oil
Trans	Hydrogenated or partially hydrogenated oils, manufactured fats found in synthetic foods

*"High oleic" means high in monounsaturated fat.

Chapter 25

Unite the Right Amount of Sodium

Sodium: Too Much Can Cause Hunger and Muscle Wasting

The recommended daily amount (RDA) of sodium is 2,300 milligrams. [156] Too much sodium can disrupt your balance of fluids, causing your kidneys and liver to work overtime to deal with the stress from the extra workload.

A 2017 clinical study published in the *Journal of Clinical Investigation* was conducted using Russian volunteer cosmonauts to evaluate the impact of controlled amounts of sodium on fluid levels. [127] Male study subjects lived in a spaceship simulator on land for 105 days, where researchers were able to completely control their food and sodium intake and measure their excretion. Keep in mind that the RDA for sodium is 2,300 milligrams. The amount of sodium given to the cosmonauts started at 6,000 milligrams per day and was increased over time to 9,000 milligrams, then 12,000 milligrams. In the first 24 hours, the participants were thirsty, and their bodies excreted the excess salt and water in their urine. Over time, however, study subjects started drinking less water and were hungrier, not thirstier.

Researchers determined that the larger intake of sodium caused the subjects' kidneys to conserve water to excrete the sodium buildup. To expel excess sodium, the body manufactures a compound called "urea." Urea is made in the liver, and unfortunately one of the ingredients of urea is nitrogen, which the body must take from muscles, causing muscle wasting. Moreover, making urea requires extra energy, which caused the subjects to feel hungry and eat more. The subjects gained fat weight and lost muscle mass. This is contrary to what you want your body to do.

A review of Elizabeth's beginning food record from Chapter 1 reveals that she was consuming over 9,000 milligrams of sodium—the mid-level of sodium being fed to the cosmonauts in the study.

Elizabeth's Food and Beverage Journal

	Beginning in October	**Sodium**	**Calories**
Breakfast	• Café mocha, 12 oz. • Plain bagel, 3.8 oz. • Cream cheese (2 Tbsp, Starbucks)	140 mg 620 mg 150 mg	290 280 260
Lunch	• Grilled chicken sandwich, • Large fries • Chocolate milkshake, medium (Wendy's)	1080 mg 570 mg 270 mg	390 530 580
Snack	• 1 Clif Bar, 2.4 oz., crunchy peanut butter • Fried mozzarella sticks, 6 oz. with 1 Tbsp Ketchup • Coke- 3 (20-oz)	240 mg 3,864 mg 154 mg 330 mg	260 1,528 19 693
Dinner	• Beef tacos, 2 • Tortilla chips, 20 with salsa • Beer, 12 oz. • Vanilla cupcake, 3.4 oz.	554 mg 238 mg 430 mg 14 mg 90 mg	400 300 52 154 350
Snack	• Kit Kat Bar, 1.5 oz. • Popcorn, 4 cups	30 mg 270 mg	218 255
Total		**9,346 mg**	6,859

Elizabeth originally consumed 9,346 milligrams of sodium a day, but according to the outcome of the study, at this level of sodium, Elizabeth, like the cosmonauts, would have unintentionally drunk less water and eaten more. With her high sodium and caloric intake, Elizabeth's body was hungry—which encouraged her to eat large amounts of synthetic foods. Unfortunately, the price she paid for the excess sodium indulgence was weight gain and muscle wasting. Not good.

The next chapter contains Nature's Food Selection Guide, which is a simplistic way to organize your foods. This systematic method of eating puts you on the path to eating real food and loving it. Nature's Food Selection Guide helps you to filter through the many food choices, allowing you to put together a working plan from nature.

Chapter 26

Unite Your Eating in a Plan

Your Plan to Consume from Nature

A good way to begin your transformation to looking and feeling better is to have a plan. Nature's Food Selection Guide makes it easy to plan meals and snacks and can help you to get into a consistent, healthy routine of eating. The plan was designed for the busy person who needs a quick guide.

In Nature's Food Selection Guide, all you have to do is select one food from each section for a meal or snack. The suggested foods in the guide are comprehensive but not exhaustive. For example, you may not see proteins you want to consume at a particular meal like breakfast, so pick a protein food off the lunch or dinner section. The foods listed in nature's plan were chosen to help you shift your cravings toward nature.

Nature's Food Selection Guide provides a range of 1,200 to 2,500 calories per day. For your specific caloric needs, use the Mifflin-St Jeor Equation in Chapter 23, then multiply the result by a physical activity level (PAL).

Nature's Food Selection Guide

Select a food from each section for every meal.

Breakfast

Protein Suggested Servings: 1–3		Whole Grain/Legume Suggested Servings: 1–3 5 or more g. of fiber	
Food	Serving size	Food	Serving size
*Cheese (soft): feta, goat, mozzarella, provolone, ricotta	1 oz	Bagel/ English muffin/ pita (sprouted-grain, whole wheat, or gluten free [GF])	1/2 piece
Cottage cheese	1/4 cup	Bread (sprouted grain, whole wheat, or GF)	1 slice
Eggs	1 whole or 2 whites	**Buckwheat/kasha, quinoa (pseudo grain) (GF) 1/2 cup	Berries: 1 cup black, blue, raspberries, strawberries, and so forth
**Nutritional Yeast	1/4 cup	Cereal or muesli (GF) 3/4 cup	Cantaloupe 1 cup
Seitan	1 oz		Cherimoya 1/2
Spirulina	2 Tbsp		
** Tempeh	1 Tbsp	Oats: (rolled/ steal cut) (GF) 1/2 cup	Cherries 15
** Tofu	2-3 oz		
Protein Powder: egg, **hemp, **pea, **soy or whey	7 g of protein per serving	Tortilla or Wrap:(6-inch, low- carb wheat, corn or GF) 1 piece	Dates 2
			Dragon fruit 1/2
			Figs 2 small

Breakfast

FRESH FRUIT Suggested Servings: 1–2		Dairy/Alternative Suggested Servings: 1		Healthy Fat Suggested Servings: 1–3	
Food	Serving size	Food	Serving size	Food	Serving size
Apple	1 small	Kefir **(Dairy)**	8 oz	Almonds	6
Applesauce	1/2 cup			Almond oil	1 tsp
Apricots	4 pieces of fruit	Milk: almond, flaxseed (alternative)	8 oz	Avocado	1/8
Banana	1 small			Avocado oil	1 tsp
Milk: hemp, oat, plant, soy (alternative)	8 oz			Brazil nuts	2
				Butter (grass fed)	1 tsp
Milk: 1% cow, goat (dairy)	8 oz			Canola oil (high oleic)	1 tsp
				Cashews	6
				Chia seeds	1 Tbsp
Yogurt: coconut, Greek, plain (unsweetened) (alternative/dairy)	6 oz			Coconut dried	3 Tbsp
				Coconut milk regular	1 1/2 Tbsp
				Coconut oil	1 tsp

Lunch

Protein Suggested Servings: 1–4		Whole Grain/ Legume Suggested Servings: 1–3	Fresh Fruit Suggested Servings: 1–2	
Food	Serving Size	Food Serving Size	Food	Serving Size
*Cheese (soft): cottage, feta, goat, gouda, mozzarella, provolone, ricotta	1 oz or 1/4 cup	Barley, Farro, Spelt 1/2 cup	Grapefruit	1/2
			Grapes	15
			Guava	2 small
**Nutritional Yeast	1/4 cup	Pasta (made with chickpeas, lentils, legumes, or whole wheat)	Kumquat Lychee Mango Melon Nectarine	4 1/2 1 cup 1 1
Seitan	1 oz		Orange Papaya Passionfruit	1 1 cup 3
Spirulina	2 Tbsp			
		Dried beans, whole lentils, peas (cooked) 1/2 cup	Peach	1 small
			Pear	1 small
** Tempeh	1 Tbsp	Bean, split pea, or barley soup	Persimmon	1 small
** Tofu	2-3 oz	1/2 cup	Plum	1 large or 2 small
Poultry (skinless): chicken, Cornish hen, duck, pheasant, turkey	1 oz	**Buckwheat/ kasha, quinoa (pseudo-grains) **(GF)** 1/2 cup	Pineapple	1 cup
			Pomegranate seeds	1/2 cup
			Prunes	3
Fish: cod, halibut, herring, mackerel, salmon, sardines, tuna	1 oz	Hummus or other bean dips (GF) 1/4 cup	Soursop	1 small

Lunch

Vegetables Suggested Servings: 3–5		Healthy Fat Suggested Servings: 1–3	
Food	Serving Size	Food	Serving Size
Artichoke Arugula Asparagus	1/2 cup cooked or 1 cup raw, or more	Flaxseed (ground)	2 Tbsp
		Flaxseed oil	1 tsp
Bamboo shoots, beans (green, Italian, wax), beets	1/2 cup cooked or 1 cup raw or more	Grapeseed oil	1 tsp
		Hazelnuts	5
Bok choy broccoli Brussels sprouts	1/2 cup cooked or 1 cup raw or more	Hempseeds	1 Tbsp
		Macadamia nuts	2–3
Cabbage, carrots, cauliflower, celeriac root, celery, chard, chervil, chives, Cilantro cucumber, daikon, Eggplant, endive, escarole, fennel, radish	1/2 cup cooked or 1 cup raw or more	Mayonnaise (made with avocado oil or olive oil, unsweetened)	1 tsp
Fermented Vegetables: kimchi, pickles, sauerkraut. Garlic, Green Beans 1/2 cup cooked or 1 cup raw, or more		Medium chain triglyceride (MTC) oil	1 tsp
Greens: beet, collard, dandelion, kale, mustard, turnip, and so forth. 1/2 cup cooked or 1 cup raw or more		Nut and seed butter 1 1/2 tsp	

Dinner

Protein Suggested Servings: 3–6	Grain/Legume or Starchy Vegetables Suggested Servings: 0–3 5 or more grams of fiber per serving	
Food Serving Size	Food Serving Size	Food Serving Size
*Cheese (hard): asiago, blue, cheddar, edam, gouda, parmesan 1/2 oz	Amaranth millet 1/2 cup Sorghum teff 3/4 cup (GF)	Breadfruit, jackfruit, soursop 1/2 cup
*Cheese (soft): feta, goat, mozzarella, provolone, ricotta 1 oz	**Soy beans (black), edamame (cooked) **(GF)** 1/2 cup	Butternut squash, sweet potatoes, yams 1/2 cup
Fish: cod, halibut, herring, mackerel, salmon, sardines, tuna 1 oz	Barley, farro, spelt	Corn, green peas, 1/2 cup lima beans
Shellfish: clams, crab, lobster, scallops, shrimp 1 oz	Legume pasta: black bean, chickpea, edamame, lentil **(GF)** 1/2 cup	Plantain 1/3 cup
		Potatoes: purple, red, medium sweet, yellow 1/2 cup
**Nutritional Yeast 1/4 cup		Pumpkin
Seitan 1 oz	**Buckwheat/kasha, quinoa (pseudo-grain) **(GF)** 1/2 cup	Root vegetables: parsnips, rutabaga, sunchokes, yams 1/2 cup
Spirulina 2 Tbsp		
**Tempeh 1 Tbsp		
**Tofu 2-3 oz		
Poultry: chicken, Cornish hen, duck, turkey 1 oz	Rice: basmati, black, brown, purple, red, wild (GF) 1/3 cup	Squash: acorn, butternut 1 cup

* Eat cheese as a condiment, not as the main protein. Limit two servings per day. (GF) = Gluten free
** Plant food that contains all nine essential amino acids, meaning they are complete proteins.

Dinner

Vegetables Suggested Servings: 3–5 *1/2 cup cooked or 1 cup raw or more*		Healthy Fat Suggested Servings: 2–3	
Food	Serving Size	Food	Serving Size
Jicama, kohlrabi, leeks, lettuce (all varieties of microgreens), mushrooms	1/2 cup cooked or 1 cup raw or more	Olives: black, green, kalamata	8
		Olive oil (extra virgin)	1 tsp
Okra, onions, parsley, peppers, radicchio, radishes	1/2 cup cooked or 1 cup raw or more	Peanuts	10
		Pecan (halves)	4
		Pine nuts	1 Tbsp
Salsa, scallions, shallots, spinach, snap peas/ snow peas	1/2 cup cooked or 1 cup raw or more	Rice bran oil	1 tsp
Squash (crookneck, spaghetti, summer, zucchini, and so forth) Spinach Sprouts	1/2 cup cooked or 1 cup raw or more	Sesame oil (high oleic)	1 tsp
		Soy nuts	2 Tbsp
Tomatoes Turnips	1/2 cup cooked or 1 cup raw or more	Seeds: flax, chia, sunflower, pumpkin, sesame	2 Tbsp
Water chestnuts, watercress	1/2 cup cooked or 1 cup raw or more	Walnut (halves)	4

For a complete meal plan that includes recipes, visit thenatureshift.com.

Nature's Food Selection Guide Calorie Breakdown

Carbs (45–55 %)
Protein (20–30 %)
Fat (30–40 %)

Food Group Specifics

Protein
(The best protein to purchase is organically grown animal/plant protein, lean, free range, and wild caught.)
Servings per day: 9–11
One serving = 35–75 calories, 5–7 grams of protein, 3–5 grams of fat, 0–4 grams of carbs

Legumes
(The best legumes to purchase are organically grown.)
Servings per day: 1–2
One serving = 90–110 calories, 3–7 grams of protein, 15 grams of carbs, 3–7 grams of fiber

Vegetables
(The best vegetables to purchase are organically grown.)
Servings per day: 5–9 (1/2 cooked or 1 cup raw)
One serving = 25 calories, 5 grams of protein, 2 grams of carbs, 3 grams of fiber

Dairy or Alternative
(The best dairy to purchase is unsweetened, hormone free, and organic.)
Servings per day: 1–2
There is a wide disparity of calories, protein, carbs, and fats depending on the type of milk chosen. Check the label for accuracy.
One dairy serving = 90–150 calories, 8 grams of protein, 12 grams of carbs, 1–5 grams of fat
One alternative serving = 25–90 calories, 1–9 grams of protein, 1–4 grams of carbs, 1–5 grams of fat

Whole Grains
(The best grains to purchase are unsweetened, sprouted, organic, gluten as tolerated, or gluten free [GF].)
Servings per day: 0–2
One serving=80–110 calories, 1–3 grams of protein, 15 grams of carbs, 5–15 grams of fiber

Starchy Vegetables
(The best starchy vegetables to purchase are organically grown.)
Servings per day: 0–1
One serving=80 calories, 2 grams of protein, 15 grams of carbs, 3–7 grams of fiber

Fruit
(The best fruit to purchase is fresh, organically grown, and unsweetened, with no sugar added.)
Servings per day: 2
One serving=60 calories, 15 grams of carbs, 3–7 grams of fiber

Healthy Fats, Oils, Nuts, and Seeds
(The best fats to purchase are organic, cold pressed, unsweetened, and unsalted.)
Servings per day of fats and oils: 3–4, nuts and seeds: 1–2
One fat serving=45 calories, 5 grams of fat

Note: The specifications I have next to each food group are not mandatory for you to follow. Please purchase whatever works best for your resources and budget.

Getting Started with Nature's Eating

Here are some tips if you need help to get started with eating real food from nature:

- o Fast and drink nothing but water for 24 hours. After your water fast, begin eating nature's foods. This will give your taste buds a reset.
- o Regularly change out synthetic foods and replace them with nature's foods. For example, if you routinely eat cookies after dinner, eat three bites of an apple before having the cookie. Then assess to see whether you still want the cookies.
- o If you cannot withdraw from suddenly eating synthetic foods, gradually decrease foods and beverages that are problematic. You will be surprised to see that after only a couple of days, you will need fewer of them to feel satisfied, and your cravings will decrease.

The Transfer Effect: How Exercise Inspires You to Eat Real Food

If you're not ready to begin a shift toward nature by eating real foods, I invite you to start with increasing your movement and exercise first. When you improve skills in one area of your life, you inescapably trigger the desire to improve in another. This is called the "transfer effect." An example of how the transfer effect works is shown in a study published in the *Journal of American College Nutrition*. When people began an exercise program, it triggered positive changes in their diet. [73] This is partly because the people in the study who made exercise a habit had greater bandwidth to practice other ways to improve themselves. When the behavior of exercise was built into their automatic conditioning, their brains were freed up to think about other things like eating better. Like the people in the study, you may find that after you start moving more, you will have an increased desire to embrace nature's foods. The next chapter touches on the second pillar of your shift toward nature: exercise.

Chapter 27

Unite Movement with Eating

Muscle Movement

To remain healthy and independent, muscle needs to be preserved throughout your life span. Just think, our primitive ancestors had to move to survive. They had to activate their muscles to acquire food by hunting and gathering, and they had to be able to escape from predators in the wild. In today's world, we survive in different ways. We can effortlessly obtain food and even have it delivered to our doorsteps, and we can make a living by sitting all day and not moving much at all. We are thankfully not running from wild beasts to keep from being eaten, but the comforts we have come at a cost. Because we aren't required to move our muscles for survival the way our ancestors had to, many adults are losing their muscle mass prematurely, causing them to partially or completely lose their independence. We are also seeing an increase in older adults becoming more disabled, experiencing more injuries related to falls, and even dying younger than expected. [118]

Inactivity has increased over time. The lack of muscle movement has been found to be an important cause of the majority of chronic diseases we see today like accelerated aging/premature death, sarcopenia (muscle wasting), metabolic syndrome, obesity, insulin resistance, type 2 diabetes, nonalcoholic fatty liver disease, heart disease, high blood pressure, strokes, cognitive dysfunction, depression, anxiety, osteoporosis, osteoarthritis, balance, bone fracture/falls, rheumatoid arthritis, colon cancer, breast cancer, polycystic ovary syndrome, pain, constipation, and gallbladder diseases. [16] Most people know someone who suffers from one or more of those ailments.

On the contrary, time spent moving your muscles in daily physical activity prevents all the diseases listed above, plus positively impacts the health of your skin, eyes, reproductive system, heart, lungs, and brain. With regular exercise, you can prevent chronic diseases, and live a life free of diseases throughout your entire life span.

Think of muscle movement or exercise as a medicine that can fix the whole body. Exercise gives you an enormous physiological health-promoting rate of return, greater than your initial outlay, and it takes up only a small percentage of your time each day. The few highlights I'll make about exercise in this book won't do it justice. I only attempt to capture the essence of the topic in hopes of communicating that a regular routine of movement is essential to help you shift your desire toward wanting more real food from nature.

Myokines

Avid exercisers notice that the benefits of exercise go beyond muscle strength. Besides increasing your ability to move around and perform daily tasks more efficiently, daily muscle movement activates repair molecules called "cytokines" (of Greek origin, *cyto* means "cell," and *kino* means "movement"), which are further classified in an internal network of chemicals called "myokines" (*myo* means "muscle"). The term *myokines* was brought into focus in 2003, [20] and to date there have now been over six hundred myokines identified. Myokines have interesting names like ghrelin, interleukin-15, myostatin, and peptide YY. [58] Outside of supporting muscle tissue, myokines support your entire system and send out anti-inflammatory messages. What scientists have discovered is that these myokines regulate your metabolism, increase angiogenesis (create more blood vessels), and increase your ability to get rid of inflammation. [63] Myokines also target hormones and other endocrine functions involved in helping you regulate your weight and blood sugar and increase your cognition. It's been found that myokines assist your body by communicating to the cells what repair or regeneration needs to be done. They also act as anti-inflammatory messengers by reducing tumor growth in major organs like your liver, bones, and fat tissue. Basically, myokines help every organ in your body. They especially assist your brain to acquire knowledge, filter through information, and increase reasoning. When you are shifting your cravings toward nature's foods, the myokines you secrete through exercise are key in helping you regenerate and adapt to new flavors.

Physical Benefits of Exercise

Apart from myokines, other hormones are released during exercise. Studies show that both endurance training and resistance training provide a stimulus to decrease the negative impacts of adiponectin and leptin—hormones that play a role in weight gain, heart disease, and metabolic dysfunction. [27] With the positive alteration of these hormones, your body is able to shift its appetites and cravings, which assist in weight control and proper eating.

Here are some other physical benefits you will enjoy from exercise:

- **Increased Mitochondrial Density**
  Remember that you have tiny powerhouses inside each of your body's cells, which are the sites where calories are made into fuel. The more muscle tissue you have, the more mitochondria you will have. Both during and after exercise, your mitochondria burn energy and lots of it. When they run out of calories, they send for help. At this point, calories are pulled from your fat cells to fuel the mitochondria in your muscles, which means you break down fat, increase your metabolism, and need to eat more calories to keep up with the demand. When you have more muscle tissue, the amount of mitochondria you have is greater. This means your body burns more calories even while you're doing something sedentary like sitting around and watching your favorite show.

- **Muscle Growth**
  When you stress your muscles through weight lifting or power

movements, microscopic tears occur. As bad as this sounds, after the tears occur, your muscles begin a repair cycle—provided that they have the right nutritional ingredients on board. This is the process your muscles use for growth. The muscle tears activate your cytokines and myokines, which go to work regenerating, building, and fortifying your muscular structure. [167]

- **Fat Loss**
The human body has evolved to preserve fat tissue needed for survival if food becomes scarce. When you exercise and enhance myokine circulation, your body receives a message that muscle, not just fat tissue, is important for survival. When the signals to maintain muscle are triggered, your body will use your fat storage to preserve muscular tissue that keep your muscles sustained. This switch is necessary for those looking to lose fat weight.

- **Enhanced Immunities**
In today's world, it's necessary to have a healthy immune system. Your immune system responds favorably to exercise. Research in the area of exercise immunology shows that moderate-intensity exercise stimulates your immune system by exchanging anti-pathogen immune cells from your circulation to your tissues. [111] Anti-pathogens fight against diseases. When you exercise, you release them into the areas where they are needed. They work to decrease and eliminate disease-causing microbes. When you exercise daily, you get a regular dose of this immune defense.

Muscle Movement and Cravings

Muscle movement or exercise assists you on your journey to eat real food and love it by reducing cravings for synthetic foods. In a small study, 11 men worked out for 12 weeks. Afterward, the men reported decreasing their cravings for synthetic foods—specifically high-fat foods, fast-food fats, and sweets. [132] This is counter to the general thought process that exercise increases cravings. The long-term effect of exercise is a decrease in synthetic food cravings, which in turn allows you to have a greater capacity to increase your cravings for nature's foods.

Exercise also helps you to eat healthfully by enhancing your moods. Brain research shows that exercise helps you decrease negative and increase positive moods. [10] In other words, if you struggle with anger, depression, or brain fog, try exercising. Exercise helps you feel better. What's more, the upbeat effects that can improve your mood right after exercise have been shown to last through the next day. [97]

Once you regularly work exercise into your schedule, you are sure to discover that the benefits of feeling invigorated and mentally stimulated for an entire day far outweigh the time it takes to exercise. If you're skeptical, give it a try. You will reduce cravings for synthetic foods, pump out positive hormones, boost your moods, increase mitochondrial density, grow muscle, lose fat, and enhance your immunities.

With all there is to gain, please make sure to put aside time every day to engage in health-promoting muscle movement and training.

Exercise Guidelines: How Much Exercise Is Needed?

To receive the benefits just listed, exercise guidelines published in *JAMA* [121] recommend that adults exercise 150 to 300 minutes (2.5 to 5 hours) a week by doing a moderate-intensity exercise like walking, water aerobics, dancing, hiking, yoga, bicycling on a level terrain, tennis doubles, or heavy cleaning, which would include washing windows or vacuuming. Or exercise for less time at a higher intensity—75 to 150 minutes (1.25 to 2.5 hours) a week if the exercise is a vigorous-intensity aerobic activity like jogging, bicycling fast or uphill, running, tennis singles, competitive sports, dancing energetically, mountain climbing, jumping rope, and so forth. The guidelines also suggest that you can combine moderate with vigorous-intensity aerobic activities. Do some or the other during the week or alternate days to stimulate your muscle tissue.

In addition to cardio exercises, increase your muscle density by doing muscle-strengthening activities like weight lifting, working with resistance bands, push-ups, sit-ups, lunges or squats two or more days a week. Also, heavy gardening, digging, and shoveling help you gain muscle.

To keep your muscles pliable, the guidelines also recommend that you work some flexibility activities into your week. The best time to stretch is when your muscles are warm. A good suggestion is to stretch after each session of exercise unless you are participating in a sport that may require specific stretches before or during it.

Another exercise recommendation, especially for older adults, is the practice of neuromotor or balance-training exercises at least two days a week. These exercises help you keep your balance as you age. Examples are walking heel to toe in a straight line, standing on one leg at a time, or standing from a sitting position.

To assess your exercise intensity, how hard you work out, a scale called the Rating of Perceived Exertion (RPE) scale was developed. Here is how to use the RPE scale. While you are exercising, mentally assign yourself a number on a scale of zero to ten. This number gauges how you're feeling during exercise. It's a simple way to assess your exertion to help you discern whether you need to kick up the intensity or ease off.

Table E shows an example of the RPE scale for both aerobic and muscle-strengthening activities and what the numbers represent.

Table E

Rating of Perceived Exertion (RPE) Scale	Aerobic Activities	Muscle-Strengthening Activities *
0	No exertion at all	No exertion at all
1 2	Very light	Very light
3 4	Light. Breathing is comfortable. You are able to hold a conversation.	Lightweight
5 6 Moderate-intensity activities	Light. You can talk, but it is difficult to hold a conversation. You are aware that breathing is harder.	Somewhat lightweight. The exercise can be used as a warmup or preparation for heavier weights.
	Somewhat hard. Breathing starts to get uncomfortable.	Somewhat hard. Weight can be lifted for at least eight repetitions.
7 8 9 Vigorous-intensity activities	Hard. You have uncomfortable, deep, and forceful breathing; you don't want to talk.	Hard. Weight can be lifted for only two to three more repetitions.
	Extremely hard	Extremely hard. Weight can be lifted for only one more repetition.
10	Maximum exertion	Absolute maximum

To see positive results, follow the guidelines in Table G.

Table G

Exercise Guidelines for Adults		
Type of Exercise	Rating of Perceived Exertion (RPE) Scale 0-10	Time per Week
Moderate-intensity aerobic activity	Light to somewhat hard (3–6)	150–300 minutes (2.5–5 hours)
Vigorous-intensity aerobic activity	Somewhat hard to very hard (7–9)	75–150 minutes (1.25–2.5 hours)
Combination of moderate and vigorous-intensity aerobic activity	Alternate light/somewhat hard (RPE 3–6) with somewhat/very hard (RPE 7–9)	150–300 minutes (2.5–5 hours)
Muscle-strengthening activity	Lightweight, somewhat hard and hard, depending on goals (RPE 4–8)	2 or more days a week
Flexibility	·	2–3 days a week
Balance-training activity (older adults)	·	2 or more days a week

With all the recommendations just listed, if it seems too overwhelming, just get started doing something. Even doing five minutes a day of muscle training or some kind of movement is better than doing zero. You can call a shortened workout your "worthwhile workout" for the day, knowing you did something as opposed to doing nothing.

Keep in mind that besides conscious exercise, you also burn some fuel by way of non-exercise activity thermogenesis (NEAT). NEAT activities—like doing the laundry, walking in a building, or wiping down a countertop—cause your muscles to burn calories, but they don't fuel your mitochondrial fires in the same way exercise does. NEAT activities are helpful for some calorie burn, but if your daily activities are repetitive, your muscles get used to them.

The next chapter touches on the third pillar of your shift toward nature—meditation. As mentioned earlier, like exercise, meditation practices help rewire your brain to embrace real food. Exercise improves your moods and assists you in enjoying foods from nature. And most importantly, to prevent you from slipping back into old eating behaviors, meditation helps you to stay focused on your journey. [50]

Chapter 28

Unite Movement and Eating with Meditation

Meditation

When you feel positive, you are able to readjust the mental and physical states that negative emotions generate. Simply put, meditation helps you feel more positive. [50] Nature's Mindfulness Meditation script is designed to help you form positive emotions toward your body and brain. These emotions fire up your desire to improve and pay attention to your own self-care. With enhanced mental health, you are better able to align your will with the desire to work toward the authentic body and brain nature intended.

The following meditation script was meant with you in mind. The transitions throughout this meditation script specifically help your mind focus on aspects of craving health. It is a mental compass toward eating real food and loving it. Before you try the meditation, you may want to get familiar with the transitions in the script.

Nature's Meditation Transition Guide

Your mind is one of your most powerful tools in shifting your cravings to nature. Nature's Mindfulness Meditation was designed to help you yoke your mind away from the external, especially food, in effort to capture your attention towards the healthy body and brain nature intended. There are six transitions to Nature's Mindfulness Meditation. Like the six nature steps, the transitions start with the letters in the word "NATURE":

> N=Notice your foods being sure they are full of nutrients to run your body.

> A=Analyze and be thankful for how the foods in nature are formed and designed to appeal to your senses of sight, smell and taste.

> T=Train your brain to see your ideal self.

> U=Unite yourself with nature.

> R=Renew your relationship with nature's foods and forgive yourself.

> E=Enjoy your journey by aligning yourself with your higher power.

The first transition in Nature's Mindfulness Meditation - Notice– reminds you to notice your foods before you eat them, being sure that they contain nutrients to run your body. Because you rely on plants and they rely on you, in this phase think of this connection and how you can increase it by eating more plants. Remember how their defensive antioxidant strategies work by donating electrons that can defend your cells against free radical damage. This is only possible when you bring nature's foods into your body. The following graphics from Chapter 2 can remind you how nature's foods contain electrons that can be donated to help prevent free radical damage.

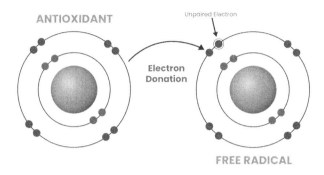

The second transition- Analyze—is designed to increase your gratitude for nature's foods. There is a reciprocal relationship between analyzing what you are grateful for and experiencing a higher quality of life satisfaction. Physiologically, when you have a sense of gratitude your heart rate decreases, and positive changes are seen in brain regions related to your emotions and motivation. [86] The second transition is designed to first shift your focus towards nature's foods and to be grateful for your food and for those who prepared it. During this transition you are encouraged to notice the colors, shapes and forms of the foods grown to nourish you. This increased awareness of plants helps you become more interested and curious about how they affect your body.

The third transition – Train—is designed to help you sharpen any dormant healthy eating skills you may already have, increase your desire for nature's foods, and see yourself living a healthy future life. In this phase you have a chance to recall any time in the past that you ate healthy foods from nature. Chances are, there have been multiple times of success in your past showing that you already have the capacity to consume beneficial foods. In this transition you can see your future ideal self at different intervals being nourished by healthy foods. Designing your best self in your mind and seeing yourself living there trains your brain to go towards that desired destination. You move towards the prize. Vividly placing your reward into your subconscious mind causes your body to work towards the reward.

The fourth transition in Nature's Mindfulness Meditation - Unite— helps you connect with nature all around you. Finding connectedness to all that is alive (including plants, animals, and people) assures your subconscious that you are not alone. Instead, you are interconnected to all life. In this phase, you are first invited to enjoy a walk outdoors and feel connected to the living world. Then, you are encouraged to surround yourself in a personal cloud of health and happiness. Your cloud will broaden and extend and allow you to slowly include more and more of what's organic—food, plants, animals, people, etc. into your cloud of health and happiness. Feeling that you are part of everything around you gives you a sense of inclusion which leads you to increased contentment, compassion and respect.

The fifth transition - Renew—is designed from the perspective that your body is talking to you. In the Renew transition you are given the opportunity to forgive yourself. By looking at what you're eating from the point of view of your body, let forgiveness flow through you, allowing yourself to let go of any past offenses, if needed.

The sixth transition in Nature's Mindfulness Meditation – Enjoy— encourages you to embrace support from a higher power or your higher self on your journey of change. Like a compass, in this phase you are encouraged to listen to the guidance of an "inner voice." This higher source is there to give you wisdom, strength and comfort. It's a force greater than yourself that can help you re-write your story and continue directing your life towards the positive. The overall mission of the Enjoy transition is for you to gain freedom and joy. This happens when nature's foods are a regular and permanent part of your life. Habitually consuming real food helps free up your thoughts so you can work on other areas of your life and reach your full potential.

Now you have a little background on Nature's Mindfulness Meditation. When you're ready to try it, sit in an upright, alert position to help you keep focused and awake, and have someone read it aloud to you. A copy of the script is available for you at Thenatureshift.com website.

Nature's Meditation Script

In this first phase, notice.

> See your body and mind being nurtured and free from harm. The minerals from the earth and the soil, insects, animals,

and sun all work together to create nutrients to help your body function at its best. See yourself bringing in nutrients from plants every time you eat.

These powerful nutrients are your personal army defending and protecting your cells.

As you bring these nutrients in, invite your memory of them to expand and see yourself looking to find them again and again.

With every bite visualize the plant nutrients preserving and protecting your body and mind.

In this next phase, analyze.

Think about how the sun sweetens the plants grown outside to delight your taste buds and give your eyes beautiful colors, shapes, and forms to see.

Think of a taste from nature that you're grateful for, a taste you experienced yesterday, last week, or sometime throughout your life span. Maybe it's the sweet taste of a berry freshly picked off the vine, the tartness of a juicy apple, or the earthiness of a crisp carrot.

Show gratitude for the abundance of flavors and varieties nature gives you.

Now, think of a person who has fed you either recently or in the past. Maybe this person bought you lunch or shared food or drink with you in some way.

Be grateful to that person for feeding you.

Analyze the abundance of food available to you and be thankful for what nature provides and for those who nurture you with food.

In this next phase, train.

> Remember the times you ate real food and how it brought nutrients into your body. These foods helped your heart pump, sending lifeblood to your entire system. As the blood flowed through your arteries, it helped your brain run, your lungs breathe, and your muscles and bones move to and from one activity to the next.
>
> You are able to keep bringing in nature's foods. You know how to do so, and when you do, the nutrients in these foods will bless you now and in the future.
>
> Know that as you continue to eat real foods, your desire for them will increase. Over time you will develop a new palate for these foods and willingly find yourself consuming more and more of them.
>
> They become what you look forward to and crave.
>
> Now, in your mind, take notice of your future self.
>
> See your body and brain as if they're performing at peak function.
>
> Notice the shape of your body in its ideal form—healthy and energetic.
>
> See how your ideal body feels mentally, physically, spiritually, and emotionally
>
> - three months from now;
> - one year from now;
> - three years from now;
> - ten years from now; and then
> - twenty years from now.

See how unique you are and see yourself bringing in the right nutrients from nature's foods to run your system. The cells that make up your body are amazing and beyond your complete understanding.

In this next phase, unite.

See yourself walking through a garden of fruits and vegetables on a sunny day.

With each breath you take in, your lungs fill with the fresh oxygen the plants in the garden freely give you. With each exhale, the plants take in the carbon dioxide you breathe out, helping them to live.

You're connected to each plant in the garden, and they're connected to you.

And as you pick a piece of fruit off the vine and take a bite, its nutrients flow into you, contributing to your body, mind, and soul.

See yourself surrounded by a circular cloud full of health and happiness.

Like a pebble being tossed onto a still lake, the water ripples into larger circles, expanding the circumference of your imaginary circle until it contains plants from nature near and far.

Then keep enlarging your circle of health and happiness to include all that's alive ten miles (16 km) away, then one hundred miles (160 km) away, then one thousand miles (1,600 km) away, then ten thousand miles (16,000 km) away until you get to the outermost circle—24,901 miles (40,075 km) away, which incorporates every living thing on the earth.

Enjoy the feeling of being connected to all that's alive on the planet and enjoy the sensation of being healthy and happy with them all.

As you build nature's foods more into your lifestyle, see your desire for them increasing.

In the next phase, renew.

Remember that wanting to feed your body well takes time and practice. Your former relationship with food, beverages, and substances is now in the past.

Listen to the message your body is giving you for the future. As you walk forward step by step, see yourself enjoying new positive actions.

Give yourself and others forgiveness. Let go of past offenses. See your body in your mind and say to yourself, "I forgive you." Allow the gift of forgiveness from your body to cleanse your mind.

In the final phase, enjoy.

Nature's food knows how to protect and care for the complex body you have. It's all in the master design. Enjoy knowing you're not alone with your struggles on your course of change.

There's a force in the universe cheering you on. It may be in the form of your future self or the God who adores you. It's supporting you as your cravings subside. This force beckons you to keep going.

Call on this power anytime you need it.

It's always there for you and wants to see you whole, free, and full of joy.

This force loves you and is kind.

With loving arms, this force embraces you and shoulders you up every time you start to droop or drift.

To close, as you're ready to close this practice, take these thoughts with you.

When you're ready, count backward from five to one. As you count, slowly wiggle your fingers and toes, shrug your shoulders, and open your eyes, feeling refreshed.

Chapter 29

Unite Summary, Recommendations, and Action Steps

Step 4: Unite

Unite Clean Eating with Exercise and Meditation to Form a Healthy, Natural Lifestyle

My "Unite" Experience

"Unite" is about joining the three pillars: healthy eating, exercise, and meditation. I can honestly say that the transfer effect I referred to earlier was true for me. Wanting to eat real food from nature happened after I started exercising. During college I took up running as a way to keep in shape. Over time I started training for races and marathons. The harder I trained, the more I paid attention to what I was feeding myself. As my health improved, I wanted to live better. Several years ago, some of my work friends introduced me to meditation. Honestly, at first I was skeptical. I thought that to understand how to meditate, I had to travel to India and spend time in a monastery, learning from monks. However, once I understood that meditation was a quiet introspective activity I could fit into my lifestyle, my faith, and a practice I could make uniquely my own, I began my day with meditation before I got out of bed. I found that meditating helped me cope with life's stressors. Now I can't imagine going through a day without tapping positively into all three pillars: meditation, muscle movement, and nourishing foods. The first two happen at the beginning of the day, and the last occurs throughout the day and evening. I'm grateful that through years of practicing, my brain and body habitually know how to do this kind of lifestyle.

Unite Recommendations

Uniting a good eating plan with exercise and meditation takes time and practice. When you put energy into improving yourself in any of the three pillars—eating, exercising, or meditating—you get good at it. The bonus is a healthier body and mind.

Action Steps for Step 4: Unite

Unite Clean Eating with Exercise and Meditation to Form a Healthy, Natural Lifestyle

A. Eat

Develop a consistent, healthy eating routine. When you regularly practice new behaviors of eating, you create healthy long-term habits. Over time your body and mind begin to crave this new way.

Nature's Eating Tips

- Consume foods and beverages throughout the day. Use one or both of these methods for spacing foods:
  1. Eat your breakfast within two hours of waking and eat every four to five hours thereafter.
  2. End your eating eight to twelve hours after you begin.

- Use Nature's Food Selection Guide to plan your meals so you can consume the right balance of foods. You can also follow an expanded meal plan, complete with recipes and a specific four-week meal plan, available at Thenatureshift.com.

B. Exercise

Engage in physical activity daily. Move your muscles regularly to build your body and help your brain both reduce cravings for synthetic foods and increase cravings for nature's foods.

C. Meditate

Cultivate a regular meditation routine. If you're new to meditation, begin with the "I Am" meditation in Chapter 26, progress to Nature's Mindfulness Meditation in Chapter 28.

STEP 5

R

Renew your positive relationship with nature's foods every day, even when you revert to old cravings.

Chapter 30

Renew your Relationship with Food

Plants work hand in hand with you to help your body and mind function, but if you don't eat them, their healing properties are of no worth.

Step 5: Renew

A. Just today, shift your focus toward synthetic foods and beverages you habitually consume and discover what they are doing for you.
B. Start small. Select one small and simple behavior you will do daily and consistently.
C. Get your support person or team together. Choose your "go-to" person or people. Everyone needs support from either one person or a team.

Elizabeth's "Renew" Journey toward Eating Nature's Foods

In Elizabeth's journey, she sometimes felt alone and isolated during the times her family indulged in fast food and synthetic foods. She temporarily returned several times to the Keto Diet. The Keto Diet allowed her to consume ample amounts of high-fat foods like bacon, cheese, and fatty meats while restricting carbohydrates. She admitted that the diet plan had worked for her in the past, and it fit more into what her family was eating; however, she always gained back any weight she had lost. After talking about how she felt the diet was restrictive, repetitive, and boring, we discussed why the Keto Diet wasn't a long-term solution for her. We also looked at ways for her to combine her eating with what her family was doing and expand her recipes to find new flavors. After failing on diet after diet, Elizabeth realized she needed to commit to eating real natural foods. Even as a highly educated professional, she was surprised to discover how confused she had been about nutrition. She assumed, as many do, that current fad diets were based on sound science and research. But she learned that most fad diets were either lacking nutrients her body needed or required her to eat foods she wasn't willing to consume for the long haul. She was ready to stay the course by seeking out nature's foods. She started observing that the more she ate from nature, the more her family slowly began to accept some of the healthy foods she introduced to them. As she found new ways to cook and make them taste good to her, she noticed this had a trickle-down effect on her family. Elizabeth and her family were increasingly eating more foods from nature.

Weight Yo-Yo

Throughout the years, I have worked with many clients who yo-yo in weight. They can lose weight, but if they fall off the wagon and return to their prior unhealthy eating habits, they tend not only to regain the weight lost but also add additional pounds. For my clients, temporarily following a diet plan isn't a sustainable approach to obtaining and maintaining long-term healthy eating habits. What I've learned is that the only way to permanently lose weight and improve your health, especially the health of your heart, is by having the desire to seek out and consistently eat nature's foods.

Even though you may not identify with having a difficult relationship with food (and I don't assume you do), you may relate to eating for emotional reasons, experiencing weight fluctuations or having episodes of uncontrolled eating or drinking. Although this book isn't about addiction or disordered eating, it's important to acknowledge unhealthy relationships that can happen with food. If you think you identify with any, know they can be addressed and unraveled. In the next few chapters, I will share some client stories, and we will look at how chemicals in synthetic foods—similar to drugs—can create hooks in your brain. Problematic eating hits everyone. We will talk about cravings and how synthetic foods can be as addictive as drugs. We'll then look at strategies for breaking free to help you renew your relationship with food. We'll also look at the stages of change and practical applications to help you embrace real foods.

Chapter 31

Renew Your Natural Opiates

Maxing Out Pleasure

When the constant consumption of sugary, fatty, and salty products continually release neurotransmitters like dopamine and serotonin, this can lead to bad habits and then addiction. Excessive neurotransmitter production, especially dopamine, impairs reasoning and causes unhealthy food consumption. In the book *The Pleasure Trap: Mastering the Hidden Force That Undermines Health and Happiness,* [22] we learned that being human, we are instinctively wired to maximize pleasure, conserve energy, and avoid pain. The ingredients in synthetic foods fit right into the pleasure-seeking trap. Just like in a drug addiction, the human brain is drawn to food to get an immediate rush.

With addiction, for most, the thought of living life without the substance seems initially terrifying. If the food stimulus is taken away, some people who have an addiction may feel like they won't be able to cope. One of my clients, who detached from a ten-year nightly ritual of drinking five to six margaritas followed by eating massive amounts of chips, shared with me that it was difficult to comprehend how she was going to live life without her evening habit. As the client worked through the process by replacing the margaritas and chips with walks with a friend around the neighborhood and took up painting as a new hobby, she broke free from the hooks alcohol, fat, and salt had on her. My client eventually discovered that life was so much better without those substances, and the corresponding peace and health brought so much more joy than the margaritas and chips ever did.

Research shows that synthetic foods, especially those with added sweeteners and fats, fit the criteria for a substance-use disorder. [54] Some signs of an unhealthy relationship with synthetic foods I've observed in my clients over the years include the following:

- There was a need for more and more synthetic foods to get the same blissful feelings they received the first time they consumed them.
- They felt that they couldn't control the food.
- They had inflated cravings for synthetic foods.
- They continued to overeat synthetic foods, even though they recognized their harmful effects.
- And/or they recognized they had a problem when they tried to stop eating synthetic foods, or if they did stop them for a while, they found themselves going back to consuming them.

The behaviors noted above indicate a harmful connection with food and beverages.

Some experts classify addiction to anything—whether it's drugs, alcohol, a device, gambling, food, sugar, shopping, tobacco, or video games—as a brain disease. [165] This means a food and/or beverage addiction may not necessarily be about the actual substance but more about the maladaptive nerve fibers in the brain. The good news is, maladaptive fibers can be rewired, especially with the right nutritional ingredients on board.

Food Addiction

Food addiction is a controversial topic because foods are made differently than drugs. Also, the type and combinations of food people eat vary and can be complex, making it difficult to track the difference between use and misuse. An addiction to a food or a number of foods can be confusing or difficult to admit. Sometimes it's tough to figure out whether you have a food addiction on your own, and for most people, even if they did admit to problem areas with food, they don't consider it an addiction. One of the hallmarks of a food addiction is denial. If you think your eating is interfering with your health and happiness, then it's time to do something about it to correct negative physical and mental effects.

The Diagnostic and Statistical Manual of Mental Disorders V (DSM-5), the fifth edition of the official text practitioners use to make psychological diagnoses, listed the criteria used to diagnose an addiction. [5] Assess yourself as you read through each criterion. See if any of them ring true for you regarding your relationship with synthetic foods and/or beverages. I've included a question at the end of each criterion to help you identify how each could be associated with a harmful relationship with a food or beverage.

1. Tolerance. The use of larger amounts or longer use: You've started to use larger amounts or use the substance for longer periods.
   Do you have a stockpile of your favorite synthetic foods?

2. Repeated attempts to control use or quit: You've tried to cut back or quit entirely but haven't been successful.
   Have you lost weight by dieting but regained the weight?

3. Much time spent using: You spend a lot of your time using the substance.
   Can you count the number of years you've been consuming the same type of synthetic foods?

4. Cravings: You've experienced cravings for the substance.
   Are you driven to eat synthetic foods or drink harmful beverages?

5. The neglect of major roles: You've failed to meet your responsibilities at work, school, or home because of your substance use.

    Have you failed to do your part at home, in the office, or with your family and friends due to your weight, poor health, or bad mood?

6. Social or interpersonal problems related to use: Your substance use has caused relationship problems or conflicts with others.

    Does your weight or health negatively impact your social or sexual activities?

7. Activities given up to use: You've skipped activities or stopped doing activities you once enjoyed to use the substance.

    Have you missed required events or social engagements so you could stay home and eat or drink whatever you wanted?

8. Hazardous use: You've used the substance in ways that were dangerous to yourself, others, or both (e.g., overdosed, drove while under the influence, or blacked out).

    Food coma?

9. Physical or psychological problems related to use: Your substance use has led to physical health problems like a fatty liver, diabetes, or psychological issues, such as depression or anxiety.

    Is your brain and body trying to tell you something?

10. Tolerance: You've built up a tolerance to the substance, so you use more to get the same effect.

    When you cut down on synthetic foods, do nature's foods taste bland? Do you constantly require more and more of your desired food or beverage to get the same sense of satisfaction?

11. Withdrawal: When you stopped using the substance, you experienced withdrawal symptoms.

    Did you have headaches, moodiness, or fatigue when you stopped eating or drinking certain foods or beverages?

Substance-use disorders are classified as mild, moderate, or severe, depending on how many of the diagnostic criteria are met. Many people identify with one or several of the criteria listed above. Please seek help if you feel you need extra support. If you feel you can do this on your own, use the NATURE steps in this book. They will help you break free from negative food habits.

Chapter 32

Renew Your Food Relationship, if Needed

Altered Relationships with Food and Beverages

In continuing the discussion about signs of unhealthy relationships with synthetic foods, I have also noticed in my clients some additional signals of problematic eating that fit into the description of either an addiction or an eating disorder.

- They plot when and where they are going to either eat or drink their favorite foods or how they will avoid them altogether.
- They purge (vomit) food or beverages after eating them.
- They eat food to enhance their mood, even though they know it is bad for them.
- They hide or sneak food or beverages so others won't see how much they are either consuming or not consuming.

In this chapter, we will look at some disordered ways of eating and how they affected some of my clients.

Anorexia Nervosa

Most often when people think about an eating disorder, they think of anorexia nervosa. Anorexia nervosa is a condition where food and beverages are purposely restricted. While it's a complicated disease with many factors involved, those who have anorexia nervosa have an abnormality in what is known as the dopamine-striatal system. [55] The striatum is a component of the basal ganglia area of the brain that helps facilitate voluntary movement. This abnormality causes a person suffering from this disease not to derive the same pleasure from eating that non-suffers experience. In fact, in anorexia nervosa, the stimulants in food and beverages that cause the release of dopamine may cause anxiety instead of pleasure.

After one client of mine was diagnosed with this disease, she confessed that her only goal was for people to leave her alone so she could be thin. My client repeated over and over to those who were trying to help (me included) that she didn't want anything else in life; the client just wanted to be left alone so she didn't have to eat. After years of hospitalizations and therapy, my client finally got well and today lives an active and productive life.

Binge Eating Disorder (BED)

Binge eating disorder (BED) was added to the DSM-5 in the 2013 edition. [42] The trait that distinguishes a BED, similar to substance-use disorder, is the loss of control. People who suffer from binge eating disorder consume foods or beverages to eliminate uncomfortable feelings like irritability, depression, anxiety, or anger. As the name implies, those with BED have regular episodes of out-of-control binge eating, as if their brains are hijacked and overtaken by automatic habits that cause them to eat large amounts of food regardless of hunger. When someone has a BED episode, the signals that come from the brain's cortex to stop compulsive eating are suppressed.

Binge eating usually happens alone when others aren't looking and is typically followed up by self-loathing. Binge eating disorder can deeply affect you and is underdiagnosed in the medical community today. I always think back to one of my clients who suffered from BED. My client described the way evenings were spent. Coming home from work, my client would drive to four or five fast-food restaurants. At each establishment, he ordered large quantities of food and drinks, ate them quickly, and then immediately drove to several more places and did the same thing.

My client described feeling "out of control" and "embarrassed about all the food he consumed." Yet despite physical discomfort, the food kept coming in, and at the end of the evening, there was a horrible sensation of guilt and shame. As we worked together, my client found healthier ways to deal with psychological pain. The more natural foods he ate and the longer we worked with each other and the doctor, the better my client felt. One day the announcement came: "I broke free from binge eating!"

Bulimia Nervosa

Those who have bulimia nervosa will binge in a similar way as those who have BED, but afterward, they will try to get rid of the extra calories in radical ways like exercising excessively, forcing themselves to vomit, or abusing laxatives. A client of mine who suffered from bulimia nervosa for years began having esophagus problems as a result of excessive vomiting. Overcoming the disease became critical to survival. As my client began seeing a therapist and started eating low-acid foods from nature like green vegetables and certain types of fruits and grains, the healing began. Over time the damage done to the esophagus was repaired, and my client was able to disassociate from the disease.

Night Eating

Binge eating can happen day or night. People who wake up from sleep and eat 50 percent or more of their calories after the evening meal and then skip eating in the morning may have a condition called night eating syndrome (NES). [2] One of my clients who suffered from NES shared his nightly ritual. My client would go to bed, get up about two hours later, prepare food, and then eat it. Typical episodes of this eating cycle occurred three to four times a night, happening in two- to three-hour intervals. My client reported being conscious and calm while eating and stated there was a peacefulness to the eating episodes. The physical consequences of night eating, however, taxed my client's heart and added a considerable amount of weight to his body. Over time and with considerable intervention with a coordinated team of professionals, he was fortunately able to disassociate with night eating syndrome (NES).

Another condition similar to NES is called sleep-related eating disorder (SRED). With SRED the person usually sleepwalks and doesn't remember eating. In one study, more than 65 percent of those diagnosed with SRED ate things that were typically inedible like buttered cigarettes or unheated frozen foods. [z]

A client of mine with SRED had her partner follow her one night and found that she had ingested large handfuls of either marshmallows or whatever candy was in the house. This behavior was unusual because my client reported that in a conscious, awake state, she didn't like sweets. Fortunately, my client was able to overcome SRED after several years by working together with a therapist and myself.

Research has discovered that hunger and sleep deprivation are two conditions that are precursors to eating behaviors that occur in the middle of the night. As with any disease, it's important to treat the root cause and seek out professional help.

Hedonic Hunger: Eating Whether You're Hungry or Not

Once stimulated by synthetic foods, your brain can drive you to consume more, regardless of whether you're hungry. This phenomenon is called "hedonic hunger" or "pleasure eating." [45] Hedonic hunger is a yearning for food despite having a full belly. It occurs mostly where tasty foods are omnipresent, like at an all-you-can-eat buffet, or in some people's homes. People with hedonic hunger have a voracious appetite, and food consumption is usually superfluous.

One of my overweight clients reported feeling helpless when at a friend's house. A celebratory cake was brought out at the end of a very large meal, and even though my client was stuffed from dinner, the cake called. My client ended up eating three large pieces of cake, stating that the sugar in the cake was so pleasurable.

The obvious consequences of hedonic hunger for my client and for everyone are weight gain and the associated diseases that occur with having too much fat weight on the body. Unfortunately, hard-earned dollars are spent to keep pleasure-seeking brains stimulated over and over and over again. Not surprisingly, despite hunger, when consumers eat food for the sheer pleasure of eating, it is a dream come true for food manufacturers.

The eating disorders just described make up a partial list of behaviors that involve food restriction and/or excessive eating. The two extremes are interrelated because they both show unhealthy relationships with foods. If you think you identify with any of the conditions listed above, please see your doctor or a therapist who specializes in eating disorders. Fortunately, with all the altered relationships with food and beverages identified in this chapter, there are remedies that help. There is healing from addiction and all disorders. Read on to find ways to break free.

Chapter 33

Renew Support

Social Connections Help You Disassociate with Substances

In 2015, Johann Hari wrote a book, *Chasing the Scream: The First and Last Days of the War on Drugs*, about his search to find answers regarding addiction. [57] He wanted to know what caused addictions and what treatment methods proved to be the most successful. In his quest, he questioned why most hospitalized patients who received diamorphine—medical heroin—didn't become heroin addicts after being released from the hospital, yet addicts living on the streets who were using less pure forms of heroin became heavily addicted.

His quest led him to fundamental research conducted over one hundred years ago when rats, while isolated in a cage and given the choice between drinking water or water laced with heroin, inevitably chose the heroin-laced water. They became addicted and eventually died.

This research formed the basic understanding of why addictions are developed; the brain directs you to seek out substances that provide a euphoric effect. If something makes you feel good, especially when you are feeling bad, you will repeat the feel-good activity, despite having undesirable consequences. Hari discovered that drug addicts were social pariahs who understandably felt an enormous amount of shame and worthlessness. Society's treatment (sending them to prison) and views toward addicts at the time (they were weak people) resulted in increased, rather than decreased, drug use. When they were in prison, their shame, isolation, and negative environments led them back to their drug-addicted lives after release. [57]

In the late 1970s, another scientific experiment on rats showed a different outcome. [3] Previously caged and isolated rats that were addicted to morphine, an opioid medication, were placed together in a spacious "rat park," where rats of both sexes were able to cohabitate and play. They had access to toys, mazes, healthy food, and most importantly, other rats. The rats in the rat park had the option of drinking water or morphine-laced water. To everyone's surprise, on the whole, the rats addicted to morphine didn't continue their addiction. They often drank the plain water and then returned to their social environment with the other rats. [3] If you translate this research to humans, it shows that imprisoning addicts isn't the best strategy for helping them recover. They need healthy connections.

Hari concluded that your brain can become addicted to the feel-good neurotransmitters secreted with positive social relationships. When addicts were in positive social and supportive environments, they didn't need the illegal drugs to make them feel good. [57]

This interesting research is also applicable to eating synthetic foods. The more you are involved in positive social interactions, the less desire and need there are to eat synthetic foods that harm your brain and body.

Get Your Partner or Team Together

One of the most important steps on your journey to renewing your relationship with food is to get support from your family, friends, or both. At minimum, choose a "go-to" person, the person you will be accountable to for reaching your goals. Find a person who will cheer you on, cry with you, and encourage you to stay the course. Everyone needs support from either one person or a team of people. Checking in to share your successes and hurdles keeps you walking toward health to refine your skills while concurrently allowing you to support others on their journey.

Chapter 34

Renew Your Reasons for Eating and Drinking

Ask: Why Am I Eating or Drinking This?

It's important to connect meaning to your actions. When you consume something you know doesn't match the big picture of what you want your life to look like, ask yourself, "What are these food and beverages like chips, cookies, candy, or alcohol doing for me?" Do you drink or eat because you are hungry and thirsty or for some other reason? If it's for another reason besides nourishment, try to consciously understand what that reason is. Then you can decide whether what you are putting in your body is worth the damage it may be causing.

An example of this approach is a habitual problem with drinking a client of mine shared. My client drank an excessive amount of alcohol at parties and consequently woke up feeling miserable the next day. Instead of recommending that my client stop drinking, I challenged him to examine his relationship with alcohol at an upcoming party. My client agreed to this approach and later reported back to me. At the party, my client had one alcoholic drink. After a few sips, he decided that the only thing he was getting out of drinking the alcohol was the ability to fit in with his friends. My client diluted the drink with sparkling water and carried it around for the rest of the evening. The friends didn't notice. My client discovered that alcohol wasn't needed to have a good time with his friends. Subsequently, my client now wakes up the following morning after parties feeling alert and refreshed without nasty hangovers.

For One Snack or Meal

You were born with a body that was meant to be fed with healthy food from nature. The healthier you are, the better able you are to bless and care for those who need you. Nature has provided you with all your body needs to be healthy and strong. Real foods from nature can help heal and nurture your body and mind, and support your immune system.

Tell yourself, "Just for today, or one meal or snack, I will shift my focus to foods and beverages that will nourish me in a healthy way." Before you consume a food or beverage, ask yourself, "What is this doing for me?" When you're conscious about what and why you're eating or drinking, you have more control over what you put in your mouth. Then try the same approach with the next snack, or carry it into the next day and the next, until your conscious decision to make good choices has transformed into subconscious, healthy habits. If you feel you may need help working through a compulsion, addiction, or eating disorder, please seek out a specialist who can help you through the process.

Chapter 35

Renew Your Readiness

There may be times when you won't care whether nature's foods are better for you. Despite their abilities to repair and heal, you want foods and beverages that will allow you to escape reality. This is when it's time to renew your relationship with nature's foods and find support for what you're trying to escape.

Readiness: From No Intention to Full-Out Action

If your health is deteriorating and you need to change the way you eat, drink, or live, then why is it so difficult? Most likely the answer is, you don't want to give up whatever gives you a rush and allows you to escape. When you're buzzed—whether it's on sugar, social media, your cell phone, caffeine, nicotine, alcohol, shopping, gambling, watching TV, street drugs, or prescription drugs—you temporarily don't have to deal with negative emotions like anger, frustration, fear, or sadness that you subconsciously dumped into your brain. Instead, you get an instantaneous pleasurable brain perk. Getting a buzz gives you an opportunity to escape, and you usually get to share the experience with others, who are eating, drinking, or doing the same things you are. It's a way of connecting.

If you use food or beverages for socializing purposes, you may say to yourself, "How will I connect if I stop getting buzzed from food and/or beverages when I go to gatherings, sports events, happy hours, parties, or dinners out?" Just as my client found that alcohol wasn't needed to enjoy time with his friends at parties, you can find joy just by being with people you care about.

Transtheoretical Model of Behavior Change

As you begin your journey, analyze where you might be on the stages of the transtheoretical model of behavior change cycle in relation to your desire to improve your health and eating habits. The transtheoretical stages of change are the following:

- Pre-contemplation: having no intention to change
- Contemplation: being aware but not taking action
- Preparation: being intent to take action
- Action: having active modification of behavior
- Maintenance: sustaining change, with new behaviors replacing the old
- Relapse: falling back into old patterns of behavior

See Figure 5 for a diagram of the stages.

Figure 5

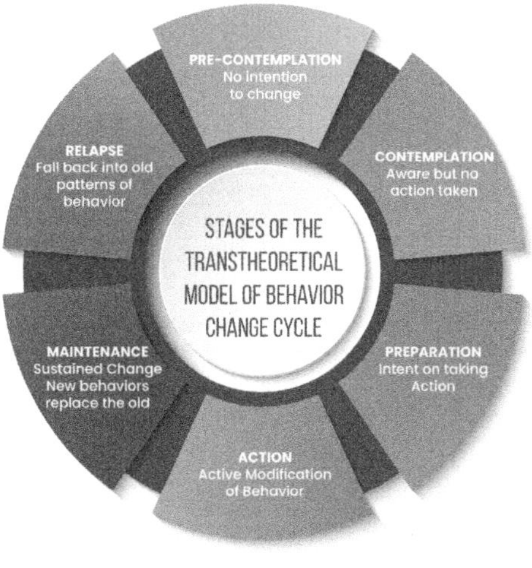

According to the transtheoretical model, you are always in a stage of change. Unconsciously you are moving forward, staying stagnant, or falling back. Behavioral change is a process that happens over time. As you adapt to changing your life to eating nature's foods, exercising, and meditating, you will muddle through the cycle and perhaps own a specific change for a while but then slip back into previously programmed behaviors.

For example, you may temporarily eat well during the maintenance stage but find yourself being lured back into eating synthetic foods. This happens all the time with foods and beverages because of the vast amounts of eating and drinking encounters you experience in your life span. The repeated behavior of consuming food and drinking beverages over time forms powerful memories webbed together by billions of previously wired nerve connections. Your brain reminds you of what it likes. In addition, your gut elicits microbial support for the foods and beverages you bring in. If you're trying to walk away from all your familiar and pleasurable delicacies in one quick swoop, you may not have given yourself enough time to develop enough healthy behaviors to replace old, destructive ones. Be patient with yourself.

Research Shows Readiness Change

Using the transtheoretical cycle above, a study was conducted that included 1,277 overweight and obese adults with body mass indexes (BMI) between 25–39.9. [78] (BMI is a measurement of a person's height and weight.) The following table shows how a person ranks:

BMI Categories	
Underweight	< 18.5
Normal Weight	18.5–24.9
Overweight	25–29.9
Obese	> 30

Participants were given a healthy eating plan with more than five servings of fruits and vegetables to help them improve their health based on their stage of change. The study was conducted for multiple behavior interventions, but one of the most surprising and interesting outcomes revealed that over 48 percent of those who began in the preparation stage with the "intent on taking action," albeit with minimal goals of eating more produce, moved into either the action or the maintenance stage at 24 months for actually eating at least five servings of fruits and vegetables a day. [78] This suggests that when you attempt to consume fruits and vegetables, you have almost a 50 percent probability of adding them to your eating for the long term.

Ready, Set, Go One at a Time

What does the change cycle mean, and how can I use it? If your health is suffering from your food and beverage choices, even if you think you cannot change, you are actually on the change cycle. This is the pre-contemplative state, in which you are weighing the pros and cons of your current eating regimen and whether changing it would improve your health. Through my personal trials and errors and my thirty-plus years of working with people, I've learned that if you want to change, you can. Trust that a journey toward nature's foods can be enjoyable and stimulating and doesn't have to feel restrictive and punishing.

If you decide to at least begin to improve your eating and enjoy real foods from nature, here are some suggestions to start you on your path: First, identify an eating or drinking habit that will lead you to habitually eating nature's foods. Choose one you're willing to tackle. Some ideas of habits that can help you embrace nature's foods are the following:

- Take time to sit and eat your meals and snacks to get more pleasure out of your food.
- Add more fruits and vegetables into your snacks and meals and taste the flavors of nature.
- Drink more water to give your body the fluids it needs to transport nutrients, run your metabolism, and maintain circulation.
- Limit alcoholic beverages to a maximum of one standard drink per day for women or two standard drinks per day for men. (One

standard drink is equal to a four-ounce wine, a twelve-ounce beer, or one-and-a-half-ounce spirits.) This practice helps you avoid toxic build-up and prevents you from overeating synthetic foods.
- Cut out or decrease synthetic foods as well as refined and white-floured (enriched) products.
- Space your meals every four to five hours to prevent blood sugar lows, which can lead to foraging for synthetic foods.
- Eat breakfast to give your body and brain energy first thing.

This isn't an exhaustive list, but it can give you a starting point. Choose one behavior to focus on at a time. Don't set yourself up for failure by trying to unravel all the automatic eating behaviors you have programmed into your brain over a lifetime. As most mothers have taught us, the most valuable things in life require work and effort on your part. And like the late American poet Robert Frost said, "The best way out is always through."

Chapter 36

Renew Summary, Recommendations, and Action Steps

Step 5: Renew

Renew Your Positive Relationship with Nature's Foods Every Day, Even When You Revert to Old Cravings

My "Renew" Journey to Loving and Craving Real Healthy Foods: Vegetables

Over 25 years ago when I was in dietetic school, we were taught about some of the phytonutrients mentioned in Chapter 2, like carotenoids, flavonoids, indoles, isothiocyanates, lignans, organosulfides, and phytosterols as well as their healing powers. Unfortunately, I found out that these health superstars were only contained in plants, not in the foods I was eating like hamburgers, burritos, and ice cream. At the time, my diet consisted mainly of synthetic foods. I didn't like vegetables, but after learning about them, I was determined to find a way to enjoy them.

I began by buying a new vegetable every week, and I combed through cookbooks, looking for tasty and healthy ways to prepare it (there was no internet then). At first, I didn't have much success. My vegetables were okay, but they left a bitter aftertaste, making it hard to buy them again.

The first time I ate brussels sprouts, I swore I would never eat them again. They tasted bitter and disgusting. I was a complete rookie in this new healthy vegetable way of eating. I had no idea how to store, prepare, cook, or enhance their flavor. However, I didn't give up. I purchased sharp knives; a large steamer; heavy-duty, stainless-steel pans; and a grill. Through trial and error, I discovered that if I steamed broccoli and artichokes just right, they were more than edible—they were tasty. Cabbage, however, was edible only if I sprinkled it with olive oil, salt, and pepper; and steamed it until it was tender but not mushy. Tomatoes were best when chopped, sautéed in olive oil with minced garlic and red wine, and cooked until they condensed. Onions, peppers, and asparagus were more flavorful when sprinkled with olive oil and sea salt and sweetened on the grill. I roasted parsnips, eggplant, and carrots in the oven until they were soft but slightly crunchy, and they were delicious. I peeled beets and cooked them in the microwave until they were soft. I also roasted beets in the oven, drizzled with olive oil and sea salt, and decided I liked them both ways.

I learned that a little minced garlic and olive oil in a skillet over low or medium heat on the stovetop is a good way to cook almost any vegetable. Initially, garlic and olive oil helped me swallow mushrooms, fresh green beans, fennel, kale, pea pods, and leeks.

As my experiments in the kitchen continued, I learned that zucchini and yellow squash are delicious when I make them into spirals (zoodles) and cook them in a tiny bit of sesame oil. Kale leaves can be rubbed with olive oil, sprinkled with garlic powder, and baked in the oven until they are crisp. I even found a way to prepare the once-dreaded brussels sprouts. I found that brussels sprouts *are* delicious if you get the small ones because they are less bitter. Slice them in half, sprinkle them with olive oil and sea salt, and roast them until they caramelize. They are labor intensive but worth the effort. I like cauliflower florets roasted in the oven or riced cauliflower (tiny pieces of cauliflower that look like rice), first sautéed in coconut or avocado oil and then cooked down with a little water until soft.

Over time, I also began to love fresh vegetables, like unpeeled cucumbers, sliced carrots, kohlrabi, and jicama. I found that salads taste best with a mixture of greens, like spinach, arugula, and dill.

Vegetables are now my favorite foods, and not only do I enjoy eating them, but I also crave them. Vegetables comprise most of my diet. For an expanded meal plan with recipes for how to cook vegetables, visit Thenatureshift.com.

Renew Recommendations

Your shift from eating synthetic foods to enjoying real nature's food doesn't happen overnight, but as you replace the bad with the good and see the benefits, it becomes easier. Establishing and/or renewing your relationship with nature's foods and beverages will take time, but the journey is worth it.

Assess how your mind and body feel daily. If you're ready for the change process, ask yourself, "Why am I consuming this?" Paying attention to why you are eating specific foods is the first step to eventually stopping them completely.

Galvanize support from family and friends or share the trip with another traveler on the same path. As with most journeys, they are a lot more impactful when shared with someone you care about.

Remember, there are phases of behavior change: not ready (pre-contemplation), getting ready (contemplation), ready (preparation), lifestyle modifications lasting for at least six months (action), and lifestyle modifications lasting from six months to five years and beyond (maintenance). Whatever phase you are in, it's okay.

Action Steps for Step 5: Renew

1. Just for today, shift your focus toward the foods or beverages you habitually consume and discover what they are doing for you.
2. Get your support person or team together. Choose your "go-to" person or people. Everyone needs support from either one person or a team.
3. Decide where you are with adding in nature's foods and write down your status on the change cycle in a notebook or in this book below.

Here's a motivational phrase you can use to help get you started. Modify it to work for you. "I am going to make this change and eat nature's foods one day at a time. I am going to give myself patience and grace throughout the process. I know this practice will take time, but the journey is worth it. Eating real food from nature will help me look and feel my best."

Write your phrase here:
_____
_____

A. Secure a support person or a small group of people to help you along your path. Write them down in a notebook or in this book below.

The person or people I am going to ask for support as I shift to eating nature's foods are the following:
_____
_____

This is what I need them to do to help me:
_____
_____

B. Ask, "Where am I on the transtheoretical model of behavior change cycle?"

Write your cycle phase here:
_____
_____

Where do I want to go next?
_____
_____

Renew Summary

Eating real foods from nature is a privilege and can be enjoyable. If you don't enjoy foods from nature now, realize their flavors can excite and stimulate you with time. Visit our company, The Nature Shift, at Thenatureshift.com and consider purchasing the meal plan. It contains recipes and cooking ideas to guide you on your path.

PART 6

E
Enjoy nature's foods as they become a permanent part of your eating routine.

Chapter 37

Enjoy Incentives

It's not about how fast you align yourself with nature; it's about experiencing the joy of nature's foods as you explore them. Let the flavors of nature entice you to want more.

Step 6: Enjoy

A. Plan Incentives

Plan daily or weekly nonfood incentives to execute your new way of eating. Redesign your incentives when they no longer excite motivation. For example, at the end of a day of eating healthily, your incentive could be to take time to read your favorite book, take a bath, or watch an episode of a guilty-pleasure TV show.

B. Share

Experiment with nature's foods, and when you begin to find healthy foods you enjoy, share them with others. Everyone can benefit from eating healthier. By sharing, you will bring in others who can help make your journey more enjoyable.

C. Make Small Adjustments

Small changes can create significant health transformations.

D. Enjoy Your Journey

There is an abundance of foods grown outdoors for you to explore. Give them a try. Have fun exploring new flavors.

Elizabeth's "Enjoy" Journey toward Eating Nature's Foods

Some foods and beverages were easy to give up, but Elizabeth admitted that she had a difficult time giving up sweets. As her palate changed, her desire for sweets dramatically decreased. She no longer ordered milkshakes or ate candy, but she found that after dinner, she wanted something sweet. To satisfy her desire for an after-dinner treat, Elizabeth indulges in a small piece of dark chocolate or another dessert but only after eating some fruit. Her favorite go-to fruit is a warm apple sprinkled with cinnamon and nutmeg and softened either in a slow cooker or microwave. Elizabeth is content with not avoiding sweets altogether and has found a way to enjoy them while also eating more healthily. To date, Elizabeth continues to nourish her body with nature's foods and beverages. She reports that she is happy with her weight and size, and she has incredible stamina and good health.

Incentives

Like Elizabeth's example, to really enjoy your path of eating nature's foods, build in some treats or incentives. Incentives can help get you motivated to stay in the change game. Some of my clients plan daily or weekly nonfood incentives to execute their new eating, exercise, or meditation plans. For example, at the end of a day of eating healthy, some of my clients enjoy time reading their favorite book, or at the end of a week of meeting their goal of eating two to four cups of vegetables every day, they explore nature or get a massage. For the other pillars, exercise and meditation, after an active week of muscle movement, some of my clients celebrate by spending extra time with a loved one or a pet. Or when they successfully do meditation five days in a row, they go see a movie with friends or watch an episode of a guilty-pleasure TV show.

Think of what incentives would get you moving and then redesign them when they no longer excite motivation. For example, maybe you tried incentives before. If, after you attempted to execute a new behavior, the habit didn't stick for long, consider finding someone *else* to give you the reward. You could ask a trusted friend to keep your reward (like a book or a new pair of workout shoes you purchased for yourself) and have him or her give you the book or shoes only after you completed your designated goal. By including another person you can trust as the holder of an incentive, you may just get the job done.

Rewards: Finding Pleasure outside Synthetic Foods

Long term rewards of consuming foods from nature seem to be intrinsic. Many of my clients who have given up eating synthetic foods state they are reaping the rewards of being able to wear stylish clothes, play with their children, and hike and bike with family and friends. Their main source of satisfaction no longer comes from synthetic foods; rather, it comes from accomplishing goals or spending quality time with their loved ones. They feel free from the habit of putting synthetic foods into their mouths for a temporary perk of dopamine and can find pleasure in other aspects of their lives. I don't know anyone who regrets eating nature's foods, but I know many who regret the negative effects synthetic foods have or had on their bodies.

Some of my more athletic clients also state that an encouraging result they get from eating nature's foods is their ability to spontaneously join others in outdoor adventures. Many report that because they are eating well, they are adventure ready when an activity emerges. They are thrilled to have good health and don't need to get in shape every time an opportunity comes up.

Others have shared the following positive outcomes:

- They have fewer annoying illnesses and feel that their immune system is able to fight off invaders more efficiently.
- They have more energy to keep up with everything on their plates and don't feel bogged down by toxins.
- They have better overall health, which allows them to participate in life.

When nature's foods are a regular and permanent part of your life and you choose them instead of synthetic foods, you are free. You choose to eat healthily because that's what you prefer. When you automatically choose nature's foods, your thoughts are free from worry about gaining weight or eating things that may harm your body. You have the certainty that what you are eating is helping you reach your full potential.

Chapter 38

Enjoy Small Steps with Age

Even a Small Change Can Make a Big Difference

When you make positive changes with your foods and enjoy their ongoing health effects, you will most likely want to continue the changes. Enjoying the change process is the best way to embrace new foods and beverages in the long run. There are some changes you will want to work out of your life and ones you will want to work in. Making even one small adjustment can bring a significant health transformation. One client of mine began the change process slowly by adding in just one cup of water a day and deleting one slice of cheese. Over time those two small changes resulted in my client's ability to lose 20 pounds and reduce his cholesterol.

Another small change that made a dramatic difference in a client of mine was adding in squats. This client had a family of young kids and an extremely busy business career but wanted to increase her muscle mass. Since she didn't have large blocks of time for exercise, she decided to do 15 squats after she used the bathroom. Her muscle was measured before she added in the squats and then two months after. Just by doing squats after she used the restroom, she was able to increase her lower body muscle mass.

As shared earlier, one small change I made in my life was to start each day with meditation. When I wake up, I mentally connect with my loved ones, express gratitude, forgive, visualize, ponder my day, and ask for support from God. This one small change takes anywhere from five to twenty minutes and has changed me. I am happier, more grateful, and more forgiving; and I feel guided in the details of my work and family life. By no means am I perfect. just ask my family, but I feel that this anchor to my day has enabled me to regularly fix what's broken in my mental attitude.

If you make your changes enjoyable and doable in any area of eating, exercise, or meditation, you will stick to them more. The important takeaway here is to do small changes suitable to you.

You're Not Too Old for Change

Permanent change with your eating happens. I have seen it in myself, my family, and over and over again in my clients. If you think you are too old for change, think again. An eighty-year-old client of mine overcame a lifelong daily habit of eating cookies with milk every night. I met my client when he was seventy-four years old, had a significant amount of weight to lose, and was battling heart disease. For the past six years, my client has been retraining his brain to choose foods from nature and has maintained the change. My client admits that the joy and energy received now after feeling healthy are far better than all the cookies that were eaten during the forty-year habit. By eating more foods from nature and giving up the nightly ritual of cookies and milk, my client lost weight and increased his stamina. This change now allows my client to have health and independence in his advanced years of life, allowing him to delay or avoid living in an assisted-living situation.

Chapter 39

Enjoy Sharing

Nature's Foods Are Best When Shared

In today's busy world, many people have a difficult time getting together with those they care about. Mealtimes can be hectic or on the go, and family dinners have stopped in many households. I remember going on a cruise several years ago with eighteen other families. We had all known each other for many years, and we had a lot of adventures on the ship and at other ports. Every night all 91 of us entered the dining room at the same time and ate our meals together. As I reflected on the cruise after it was over, I can honestly say that being together in the dining room was my favorite part of the cruise. Also, in 2020 and 2021, during the pandemic when all Californians were ordered to "shelter in place" to avoid the spread of the coronavirus (COVID-19), our family sat down every night for meals. Eating together made the pandemic bearable. Sitting and eating dinner became a ritualistic bond that gave us all a place to feel connected and secure during a bizarre time.

Whenever you can share nature's foods with others, I invite you to do so. Eating and drinking together creates bonds. People in all cultures worldwide congregate to enjoy meals. As you experiment with nature's foods and find combinations of healthy foods you enjoy, share them. Sharing can happen in all phases of a food's life cycle, from growing it, picking it, prepping it, cooking it, and then eating it. Everyone can benefit from seeing the process food goes through before it ends up in his or her mouth. I remember once hearing this simple phrase: "People who grow kale eat kale." Once you take the step to embrace nature's food in any phase, share your experience. By sharing, you will bring in others who can help make your journey more enjoyable.

"Colby's Enjoy Journey" is a story a client I worked with years ago shared with me. His story illustrates how the change process from consuming synthetic foods to desiring nature's foods changed not only his life for the better but also the life of a loved one.

Colby's Enjoy Journey

Colby always felt tired, so he routinely slept in as late as possible in the mornings, giving himself just barely enough time to shower and make it to high school on time. He either skipped breakfast or ate a piece of toast while heading out the door. During his morning break, he hit the vending machine and grabbed a bag of chips. At lunchtime, he and his football buddies drove to the local fast-food restaurant and ate a couple of cheeseburgers with bacon, a large fries, and a chocolate shake. All the guys were eating like that, and since Colby was a defensive player on the team, it was natural that he would fill his large, overweight frame with these same foods.

What Colby felt, however, was a sense of isolation and emptiness. Although he had eaten a huge lunch, he wasn't satisfied, and he wanted more and wondered why. The desire to eat synthetic food was so compelling that Colby couldn't wait to eat again. His family's pantry was filled with cookies, chips, candy, and soda; and he spent his afternoons consuming them.

Fortunately, Colby liked to cook and helped his mom or dad make dinner. Regular family meals were pasta or potatoes and meat. If there were vegetables, they typically came from the freezer or a can. Since Colby didn't like the taste of vegetables, he frequently skipped them. After-dinner snacking while watching television was a nightly family habit.

During his high school years, Colby frequently had stomachaches, headaches, and low energy. But he didn't equate his diet with his symptoms. He thought they were due to the stress of his life as a teenager.

Colby went on to college, where he met and married Emily, the love of his life. Emily and Colby often spent evenings making cookie dough and eating half the dough before it even made it into the oven. Then they ended up eating all the warm cookies as soon as they came out. Over time, Colby physically began to associate feeling bad with a high sugar intake. He felt ill from the nightly sugar overload. Eventually, Colby and Emily concluded that they wanted to lose weight and feel better. However, they had tried diets in the past, but none had worked permanently. He always returned to his bad eating habits.

At the point where Colby desperately wanted to feel better, he and Emily decided to quit processed sugar and see what life would be like. They substituted the sugar they ate with food from nature.

That was many years ago.

Now when Colby's alarm clock sounds, he rolls over, gives Emily a kiss, and heads to the kitchen. Breakfast still isn't a big meal, but since he's committed to eating breakfast, he frequently starts his day with a protein shake. For lunch, Colby eats a large pile of green, leafy vegetables with legumes and several glasses of water. He snacks on carrots and protein foods like hard-boiled eggs. For dinner, Colby and Emily create dishes with lots of vegetables and fresh cuts of organically grown meat. Since Colby likes to cook, he and Emily enjoy making new, tasty recipes using fresh herbs and spices. The adventure of trying new foods has become a new hobby. Colby and Emily now spend their evenings either going for a walk or doing something active. Colby states that he feels more energetic and is no longer obsessed with eating synthetic foods. He feels that he is finally giving his body what it needs and is enjoying the health benefits.

Colby experienced a paradigm shift with food. He moved away from thinking about synthetic foods all the time and feeling lethargic and sick to desiring food and beverages that made his mind and body feel great. Now with sugar out of his system, Colby has clarity and the ability to make better food choices. When asked whether he misses the nightly cookies, Colby replies, "Nah." He has no urge or desire to go back to the cookie dough lifestyle. And with Emily by his side, the two of them will be living with clarity and health for the rest of their lives.

Chapter 40

Enjoy Summary, Recommendations, and Action Steps

My "Enjoy" Experience: Putting It All Together

Throughout my journey to discover why I and others I knew had learned to eventually enjoy nature's foods after previously disliking them, I concluded that adapting to nature's foods and beverages was a multistep progression. Desiring to eat nature's foods didn't happen the first time I ate a vegetable. The process went something like this:

First, my prefrontal cortex (logical, rational) part of my brain decided I should eat nature's foods and beverages after studying their amazing health benefits. I began to notice and analyze the differences between synthetic foods and nature's foods and how I felt after eating each type of food. I found that cognitively I could associate how eating and drinking from nature affected my mind and body positively but only if I was in the right frame of mind and free from stress. Routine exercise enabled me to secrete the right hormones and brain chemicals, which helped to lower my stress, change my appetite, and build more muscle. For me timing was important. When my life had periods of calmness, I began introducing nature's foods one at a time until I was enjoying them. This practice trained my brain to crave new foods because I was consistently eating them. I then combined nature's way of eating with exercise and meditation, and I developed a much healthier lifestyle. I felt like I was developing a renewed relationship with nature. My gut microbiome must have liked the fibrous foods I was bringing in because I noticed a dramatic decrease in illnesses. I was most likely securing an army of helpful security guards, who helped build and strengthen my immune system.

Other than a cold once in a while, I feel healthy. I stopped having frequent bladder and kidney infections, which I had been previously prone to. I feel like something is encouraging me to desire and then crave nature's foods, because it's not a struggle for me to eat them. Figure 6 outlines my journey toward nature's foods and the health, fitness, and energy I enjoy today. This is a path anyone can take—and that includes you.

Figure 6

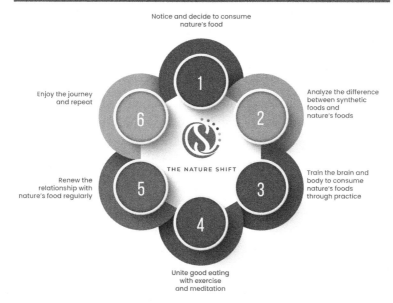

Today, an external prompt for me to consume nature's bounty is the sweet smell of vegetables roasting in the oven after they have caramelized and are almost ready to eat. Internally, I am cued (I assume) by the microbes in my gut signaling my brain to find more of them. After I eat vegetables or other kinds of nature's foods and beverages, I must be creating positive memories because I want to eat more of them. The benefits? *Besides enjoying incredible health, one unexpected benefit I have received from eating fresh foods from nature is that I feel closer to the Creator who made them for me. I now have a deep sense of gratitude for nature's foods because I believe these foods were carefully designed for the health and longevity of my body and your body.*

Your Change

Since you have read this far, you probably desire to make a change and start the process of craving foods and beverages from nature. Just think. One day you may find yourself answering the question posed at the beginning of the book—Which is healthier, a carrot or a cheese puff?—with your own question: Why would I choose a cheese puff if I crave a carrot? No matter your age, you can always make a change toward nature and receive its benefits. Whenever it feels comfortable, know that nature is patiently waiting to nourish and give you its protective and healing powers.

While you are shifting your cravings, pay attention to what is going right. Acknowledge the improvements you're making and be patient with yourself. The process of change takes time. As mentioned earlier, shifting your cravings can take two years or longer.

Enjoy Action Plan

Plan daily or weekly nonfood incentives for executing your new eating, exercise, or meditation plan. Redesign your incentives when they no longer excite motivation. Write down your incentives in a notebook or in this book below.

My daily nonfood incentive for eating nature's foods is

___

When this incentive no longer motivates me, I will use this daily nonfood incentive instead:

___

My weekly nonfood incentive for exercise is

___

When this incentive no longer motivates me, I will use this weekly nonfood incentive instead:

___

My weekly nonfood incentive for meditation is

___

When this incentive no longer motivates me, I will use this weekly nonfood incentive instead:

___

Eat Real Food and Love It
Nature Step Summary

Notice the foods you are eating each day.

- Gather data: pay attention to and record what you are currently eating and drinking.

Analyze the contents of the foods you eat before putting them in your body.

- Analyze the ingredients on a packaged food label. Learn about what you are eating.
- Analyze how close your food and beverages are to nature. Be certain that you can find your food in nature.

Train your brain to form new positive connections with nature's foods.

- Train your thoughts and visualize your future self enjoying nature's foods. See yourself eating and drinking real food from nature.
- Practice: learning to seek foods from nature takes practice.
- Regularly do mindfulness and meditation to manage stress. Practice and/or expand your meditation and stress management techniques.

Unite clean eating with exercise and meditation to form a healthy, natural lifestyle.

- Eating: develop a consistent, healthy eating routine. Use Nature's Food Selection Guide to plan your meals and consume the right balance of foods.
- Exercise: move regularly to build your body and help your brain reduce cravings.
- Meditation: cultivate a regular, meditation routine.

Renew your positive relationship with nature's foods every day, even when you revert to old cravings.

- Shift your Focus. Discover what your foods are doing for you.
- Start small. Select one small, simple behavior you will do regularly and consistently.
- Get your support person or team together. Everyone needs support.

Enjoy nature's foods as they become a permanent part of your eating routine.

- Incentives: plan nonfood incentives.
- Share: bring in others to help make your journey more enjoyable.
- Make small adjustments. Small changes can create significant health transformations.
- Enjoy your journey. Have fun exploring new flavors.

Enjoy Your Path

By changing your focus to eating fresh foods from nature, you can live healthier. Your body will be well maintained by all the phytonutrients coming in. When you crave foods from nature, your energy levels increase, while your health concerns decrease. Through perseverance, your optimal health and wellness can be obtained. Nature is and always has been calling you to align your body, mind, and soul with its goodness. And as a gift for eating nature's foods, you will function at full capacity and increase your innate potential to live a free, independent, and incredible life.

To find support on your path to eating real food and to find meal plans and recipes, visit The Nature Shift at the following:
- Website: Thenatureshift.com
- Email: iamhealthy@thenatureshift.com
- Instagram: @the.nature.shift
- Facebook: @thenatureshift

References

1. Alberini, C. M., and E. R. Kandel. 2015. "The Regulation of Transcription in Memory Consolidation." *Cold Spring Harbor Perspectives in Biology* 7 (1): 2-3. https://doi.org/10.1101/cshperspect.a021741.

2. Alberts, B., A. Johnson, J. Lewis, M. Raff, K. Roberts, and P. Walter. 2002. *Molecular Biology of the Cell*. 4th edition. New York: Garland Science; The RNA World and the Origins of Life. Available from ncbi.nlm.nih.gov/books/NBK26876/.

3. Alexander, B. K., R. B. Coambs, and P. F. Hadaway. 1978. "The Effect of Housing and Gender on Morphine Self-Administration in Rats." *Psychopharmacology* 58 (2): 175–179. https://doi.org/10.1007/BF00426903.

4. Allison, A., and A. Fouladkhah. 2018. "Adoptable Interventions, Human Health, and Food Safety Considerations for Reducing Sodium Content of Processed Food Products." *Foods* 7 (2): 16. https://doi.org/10.3390/foods7020016.

5. American Psychiatric Association. *Diagnostic and Statistical Manual of Mental Disorders*. Fifth Edition. Arlington, VA American Psychiatric Association, 2013: 483-487. https://dsm.psychiatryonline.org/doi/book/10.1176/appi.books.9780890425787.

6. Arya, S. S., A. R. Salve, and S. Chauhan. 2016. "Peanuts as Functional Food: A Review." *Journal of Food Science and Technology* 53 (1): 31–41. https://doi.org/10.1007/s13197-015-2007-9.

7. Auger, R. R. 2006. "Sleep-Related Eating Disorders." *Psychiatry* 3 (11): 64–70. https://pubmed.ncbi.nlm.nih.gov/20877520/.

8. Ayaz, M., A. Sadiq, M. Junaid, F. Ullah, M. Ovais, I. Ullah, J. Ahmed, and M. Shahid. 2019. "Flavonoids as Prospective Neuroprotectants and Their Therapeutic Propensity in Aging Associated Neurological Disorders." *Frontiers in Aging Neuroscience* 11: 155. https://doi.org/10.3389/fnagi.2019.00155.

9. Baraldi, L. G., E. Martinez Steele, D. S. Canella, and C. A. Monteiro. 2018. "Consumption of Ultra-Processed Foods and Associated Sociodemographic Factors in the USA between 2007 and 2012: Evidence from a Nationally Representative Cross-Sectional Study." *BMJ Open* 8 (3): e020574. ncbi.nlm.nih.gov/pmc/articles/PMC5855172/.

10. Basso, J. C., and W. A. Suzuki. 2017. "The Effects of Acute Exercise on Mood, Cognition, Neurophysiology, and Neurochemical Pathways: A Review." *Brain Plasticity* 2 (2): 127–152. https://doi.org/10.3233/BPL-160040.

11. Berg, J. M., J. L. Tymoczko, and L. Stryer. 2002. "Food Intake and Starvation Induce Metabolic Changes." *Biochemistry*. 5th ed. New York: W H Freeman. Section 30.3. 1264-1269. Accessed May 28, 2022. https://biokamikazi.files.wordpress.com/2013/10/biochemistry-stryer-5th-ed.pdf.

12. Berke, J. D. 2018. "What Does Dopamine Mean?" *Nature Neuroscience* 21 (6): 787–793. https://doi.org/10.1038/s41593-018-0152-y.

13. Bik, E. M., J. A. Ugalde, J. Cousins, A. D. Goddard, J. Richman, and Z. S. Apte. 2018. "Microbial Biotransformations in the

Human Distal Gut." *British Journal of Pharmacology* 175 (24): 4404–4414. https://doi.org/10.1111/bph.14085.

14. Bodenlos, J. S., K. L. Schneider, J. Oleski, K. Gordon, A. J. Rothschild, and S. L. Pagoto. 2014. "Vagus Nerve Stimulation and Food Intake: Effect of Body Mass Index." *Journal of Diabetes Science and Technology* 8 (3): 590–595. https://doi.org/10.1177/1932296814525188.

15. Bollet, A. J. 1992. "Politics and Pellagra: The Epidemic of Pellagra in the U.S. in the Early Twentieth Century." *Yale J Biol Med.* 65 (3): 211–21. https://www.ncbi.nlm.nih.gov/pubmed/1285449.

16. Booth, F. W., C. K. Roberts, and M. J. Laye. 2012. "Lack of Exercise Is a Major Cause of Chronic Diseases." *Comprehensive Physiology* 2 (2): 1143–1211. https://doi.org/10.1002/cphy.c110025.

17. Breit, S., A. Kupferberg, G. Rogler, and G. Hasler. 2018. "Vagus Nerve as Modulator of the Brain-Gut Axis in Psychiatric and Inflammatory Disorders." *Frontiers in Psychiatry* 9: 44. https://doi.org/10.3389/fpsyt.2018.00044.

18. Breslin, P. A. 2013. "An Evolutionary Perspective on Food and Human Taste." *Current Biology* 23 (9): R409–R418. https://doi.org/10.1016/j.cub.2013.04.010.

19. Burdock G. 2007. "Safety Assessment of Castoreum Extract as a Food Ingredient." *Int J Toxicol* 26 (1): 51–55. Accessed May 17, 2020. https://doi.org/10.1080/10915810601120145.

20. Bylund, A., N. Saarinen, J. X. Zhang, A. Bergh, A. Widmark, A. Johansson, E. Lundin, H. Adlercreutz, G. Hallmans, P. Stattin, and S. Mäkela. 2005. "Anticancer Effects of a Plant Lignan 7-Hydroxymatairesinol on a Prostate Cancer Model in Vivo." *Experimental Biology and Medicine* 230 (3): 217–223. https://doi.org/10.1177/153537020523000308.

21. Camina, E., and F. Güell. 2017. "The Neuroanatomical, Neurophysiological and Psychological Basis of Memory: Current Models and Their Origins." *Frontiers in Pharmacology* 8: 438. https://doi.org/10.3389/fphar.2017.00438.

22. Cantwell, M., and C. Elliott. 2017. "Nitrates, Nitrites and Nitrosamines from Processed Meat Intake and Colorectal Cancer Risk." *Journal of Clinical Nutrition & Dietetics* 3 (4): 27. https://clinical-nutrition.imedpub.com/nitrates-nitrites-and-nitrosamines-from-processed-meat-intake-and-colorectalcancer-risk.pdf.

23. Carmel, R. 2005. "Folic acid." In Shils, M., M. Shike, A. Ross, B. Caballero, and R. J. Cousins, eds. *Modern Nutrition in Health and Disease.* 11th ed. Baltimore, MD: Lippincott Williams & Wilkins, 470–81. https://treatment.tbzmed.ac.ir/uploads/User/47/nutrition/1394/modern%20nutrition.pdf.

24. Casselbury, K. 2018. "The Average Fat Intake of SAD." Accessed May 25, 2020. https://healthyeating.sfgate.com/average-fat-intake-sad-11370.html.

25. Chamberlain, S. R., U. Müller, A. D. Blackwell, L. Clark, T. W. Robbins, and B. J. Sahakian. 2006. "Neurochemical Modulation of Response Inhibition and Probabilistic Learning in Humans." *Science* 311 (5762): 861–863. https://www.ncbi.nlm.nih.gov/pmc/articles/PMC1867315/.

26. Childs, C. E., P. C. Calder, and E. A. Miles. 2019. "Diet and Immune Function." *Nutrients* 11 (8): 1933. https://doi.org/10.3390/nu11081933.

27. Clark, J. E. 2015. "Diet, Exercise or Diet with Exercise: Comparing the Effectiveness of Treatment Options for Weight-Loss and Changes in Fitness for Adults (18–65 Years Old) Who Are Overfat, or Obese; systematic review and meta-analysis."

Journal of Diabetes & Metabolic Disorders 14: 31. https://doi.org/10.1186/s40200-015-0154-1.

28. Cohen, P., and B. M. Spiegelman. 2016. "Cell Biology of Fat Storage." *Molecular Biology of the Cell* 27 (16): 2523–2527. https://doi.org/10.1091/mbc.E15-10-0749.

29. Collins, G. 1994. "Pepsico Pushes a Star Performer." *New York Times*. Accessed May 26, 2020. https://www.nytimes.com/1994/11/03/business/pepsico-pushes-a-star-performer.html.

30. Crider, K. S., L. B. Bailey, and R. J. Berry. 2011. "Folic Acid Food Fortification—Its History, Effect, Concerns, and Future Directions." *Nutrients* 3 (3): 370–384. https://doi.org/10.3390/nu3030370.

31. Costantini, A., E. Trevi, M. I. Pala, and R. Fancellu. 2016. "Can Long-Term Thiamine Treatment Improve the Clinical Outcomes of Myotonic Dystrophy Type 1?" *Neural Regeneration Research* 11 (9): 1487–1491. https://doi.org/10.4103/1673-5374.191225.

32. Courchesne-Loyer, A., E. Croteau, C. A. Castellano, V. St-Pierre, M. Hennebelle, and S. C. Cunnane. 2017. "Inverse Relationship between Brain Glucose and Ketone Metabolism in Adults during Short-Term Moderate Dietary Ketosis: A Dual Tracer Quantitative Positron Emission Tomography Study." *Journal of Cerebral Blood Flow and Metabolism: Official Journal of the International Society of Cerebral Blood Flow and Metabolism* 37 (7): 2485–2493. https://doi.org/10.1177/0271678X16669366.

33. Culp-Ressler, T. 2014. "How Food Companies Trick You into Thinking You're Buying Something Healthy." *Think Progress*. Accessed May 16, 2020. https://thinkprogress.org/how-food-companies-trick-you-into-thinking-youre-buying-something-healthy-4b5c3cc960b/.

34. Dariush, M., R. Irwin, and U. Ricardo. 2018. "History of Modern Nutrition Science—Implications for Current Research, Dietary Guidelines, and Food Policy." *BMJ* 361: k2392. https://doi.org/10.1136/bmj.k2392.

35. De la Monte, S. M., and M. Tong, 2009. "Mechanisms of Nitrosamine-Mediated Neurodegeneration: Potential Relevance to Sporadic Alzheimer's Disease." *Journal of Alzheimer's Disease* 17 (4): 817–825. https://doi.org/10.3233/JAD-2009-1098.

36. Delli Bovi, A. P., L. Di Michele, G. Laino, and P. Vajro. 2017. "Obesity and Obesity Related Diseases, Sugar Consumption and Bad Oral Health: A Fatal Epidemic Mixtures: The Pediatric and Odontologist Point of View." *Translational Medicine @ UniSa* 16: 11–16. https://www.ncbi.nlm.nih.gov/pmc/articles/PMC5536157/.

37. Dhaka, V., N. Gulia, K. S. Ahlawat, and B. S. Khatkar. 2011. "Trans Fats—Sources, Health Risks and Alternative Approach - A Review." *Journal of Food Science and Technology* 48 (5): 534–541. https://doi.org/10.1007/s13197-010-0225-8.

38. "Dietary Reference Intakes (DRIs): Acceptable Macronutrient Distribution Ranges." 2002/2005. Accessed September 2, 2020. https://www.ncbi.nlm.nih.gov/books/NBK56068/table/summarytables.t5/?report=objectonly.

39. DiNicolantonio, J. J., and J. H. OKeefe. 2017. "Added Sugars Drive Coronary Heart Disease via Insulin Resistance and Hyperinsulinemia: A New Paradigm." *Open Heart* 4 (2): e000729. https://doi.org/10.1136/openhrt-2017-000729.

40. DiNicolantonio, J. J., and J. H. O'Keefe. 2018. "Importance of Maintaining a Low Omega-6/Omega-3 Ratio for Reducing Inflammation." *Open Heart* 5 (2): e000946. https://doi.org/10.1136/openhrt-2018-000946.

41. Drexler, M. 2010. "How Infection Works. What You Need to Know about Infectious Disease." Institute of Medicine (US). Washington (DC): National Academies Press (US). https://www.ncbi.nlm.nih.gov/books/NBK209710/.

42. Ely, A. V., and A. Cusack. 2015. "The Binge and the Brain." *Cerebrum: The Dana Forum on Brain Science*, cer-12-15. https://www.ncbi.nlm.nih.gov/pmc/articles/PMC4919948/.

43. Engelen, L., R. A. de Wijk, J. F. Prinz, A. M. Janssen, H. Weenen, and F. Bosman. 2003. "The Effect of Oral and Product Temperature on the Perception of Flavor and Texture Attributes of Semi-Solids." *Appetite* 41 (3): 273–281. https://doi.org/10.1016/s0195-6663(03)00105-3.

44. Erbsloh, F., A. Bernsmeier, and H. Hillesheim. 1958. "The Glucose Consumption of the Brain and Its Dependence on the Liver." *Archiv fur Psychiatrie und Nervenkrankheiten, Vereinigt mit Zeitschrift fur Die Gesamte Neurologie und Psychiatrie* 196 (6): 611–626. https://pubmed.ncbi.nlm.nih.gov/13534602/.

45. Espel-Huynh, H. M., A. F. Muratore, and M. R. Lowe. 2018. "A Narrative Review of the Construct of Hedonic Hunger and Its Measurement by the Power of Food Scale." *Obesity Science and Practice* 4 (3): 238–249. https://doi.org/10.1002/osp4.161.

46. Esselstyn, C. B. 2017. "A Plant-Based Diet and Coronary Artery Disease: A Mandate for Effective Therapy." *Journal of Geriatric Cardiology* 14 (5): 317–320. https://www.ncbi.nlm.nih.gov/pmc/articles/PMC5466936/.

47. FEMA. n.d. "Where Do Flavors Come From?" Accessed August 21, 2022. https://www.femaflavor.org/flavors-come.

48. Fernández-Elías, V. E., J. F. Ortega, R. K. Nelson, and R. Mora-Rodriguez. 2015. "Relationship between Muscle Water and Glycogen Recovery after Prolonged Exercise in the Heat in

Humans." *European Journal of Applied Physiology* 115 (9): 1919–1926. https://doi.org/10.1007/s00421-015-3175-z.

49. Forouhi, N. G., R. M. Krauss, G. Taubes, and W. Willett. 2018. "Dietary Fat and Cardiometabolic Health: Evidence, Controversies and Consensus for Guidance." *BMJ* 361: k2139. https://doi.org/10.1136/bmj.k2139.

50. Fredrickson, B. L., A. J. Boulton, A. M. Firestine, P. Van Cappellen, S. B. Algoe, M. M. Brantley, S. L. Kim, J. Brantley, and S. Salzberg. 2017. "Positive Emotion Correlates of Meditation Practice: A Comparison of Mindfulness Meditation and Loving-Kindness Meditation." *Mindfulness* 8 (6): 1623–1633. https://doi.org/10.1007/s12671-017-0735-9.

51. Gardner, B., P. Lally, and J. Wardle, 2012. "Making Health Habitual: the Psychology of 'Habit-Formation' and General Practice." *British Journal of General Practice: The Journal of the Royal College of General Practitioners* 62 (605): 664–666. https://doi.org/10.3399/bjgp12X659466.

52. Gasperi, V., M. Sibilano, I. Savini, and M. V. Catani. 2019. "Niacin in the Central Nervous System: An Update of Biological Aspects and Clinical Applications." *International Journal of Molecular Sciences* 20 (4): 974. https://doi.org/10.3390/ijms20040974.

53. Gaynor, P., R. Bonnette, E. Garcia Jr., L. Kahl, and L. Valerio Jr. 2006. "FDA's Approach to the GRAS Provision: A History of Processes." Excerpted from Poster Presentation at the FDA Science Forum, April 2006. US Food and Drug Administration. Accessed May 16, 2020. https://www.fda.gov/food/generally-recognized-safe-gras/fdas-approach-gras-provision-history-processes.

54. Gordon, E. L., A. H. Ariel-Donges, V. Bauman, and L. J. Merlo. 2018. "What Is the Evidence for 'Food Addiction?' A Systematic Review." *Nutrients* 10 (4): 477. https://doi.org/10.3390/nu10040477.

55. Gorwood, P., C. Blanchet-Collet, N. Chartrel, J. Duclos, P. Dechelotte, M. Hanachi, S. Fetissov, N. Godart, J-C Melchior, N. Ramoz, C. Rovere-Jovene, V. Tolle, O. Viltart, and J. Epelbaum on behalf of the GIR-AFDAS-TCA Group. 2016. "New Insights in Anorexia Nervosa." *Frontiers in Neuroscience* 10: 256. https://www.frontiersin.org/articles/10.3389/fnins.2016.00256/full.

56. Guyer, L., S. S. Hofstetter, B. Christ, B. S. Lira, M. Rossi, and S. Hörtensteiner. 2014. "Different Mechanisms Are Responsible for Chlorophyll Dephytylation during Fruit Ripening and Leaf Senescence in Tomato." *Plant Physiology* 166 (1): 44–56. https://doi.org/10.1104/pp.114.239541.

57. Hari, J. 2015. *Chasing the Scream: The First and Last Days of the War on Drugs*. 1st ed. New York: Bloomsbury USA. https://www.bloomsbury.com/us/chasing-the-scream-9781620408902/.

58. He, Z., Y. Tian, P. L. Valenzuela, C. Huang, J. Zhao, P. Hong, Z. He, S. Yin, and A. Lucia. 2018. "Myokine Response to High-Intensity Interval vs. Resistance Exercise: An Individual Approach." *Front. Physiol.* 9: 1735. https://doi.org/10.3389/fphys.2018.01735.

59. Heaven, Michael, and David Nash. 2012. "Recent Analyses Using Solid Phase Microextraction in Industries Related to Food Made into or from Liquids." *Food Control* 27 (1): 214–227. http://dx.doi.org/10.1016/j.foodcont.2012.03.018.

60. Hibbard, B. M., E. D. Hibbard, and T. N. Jeffcoate. 1965. "Folic Acid and Reproduction." *Acta obstetricia et gynecologica Scandinavica* 44 (3): 375–400. https://doi.org/10.3109/00016346509155874.

61. Hibbing, M. E., C. Fuqua, M. R. Parsek, and S. B. Peterson. 2010. "Bacterial Competition: Surviving and Thriving in the Microbial Jungle." Nature Reviews. *Microbiology* 8 (1): 15–25. https://doi.org/10.1038/nrmicro2259.

62. Higdon, J. V., B. Delage, D. E. Williams, and R. H. Dashwood. 2007. "Cruciferous Vegetables and Human Cancer Risk: Epidemiologic Evidence and Mechanistic Basis." *Pharmacological Research* 55 (3): 224–236. https://doi.org/10.1016/j.phrs.2007.01.009.

63. Hoffmann, C., and C. Weigert. 2017. "Skeletal Muscle as an Endocrine Organ: The Role of Myokines in Exercise Adaptations." *Cold Spring Harbor Perspectives in Medicine* 7 (11): a029793. https://doi.org/10.1101/cshperspect.a029793.

64. Hölzel, B. K., S. W. Lazar, T. Gard, Z. Schuman-Olivier, D. R. Vago, and U. Ott. 2011. "How Does Mindfulness Meditation Work? Proposing Mechanisms of Action from a Conceptual and Neural Perspective." *Perspectives on Psychological Science: A Journal of the Association for Psychological Science* 6 (6): 537–559. https://doi.org/10.1177/1745691611419671.

65. How Products Are Made. n.d. "Cheese Curl." Accessed April 25, 2020. http://www.madehow.com/Volume-5/Cheese-Curl.html.

66. Ibi, D., F. Suzuki, and M. Hiramatsu. 2018. "Effect of AceK (acesulfame potassium) on Brain Function under Dietary Restriction in Mice." *Physiology & Behavior.* 188 (1): 291–297. https://doi.org/10.1016/j.physbeh.2018.02.024.

67. InformedHealth.org. 2011. "How Does Our Sense of Taste Work?" Institute for Quality and Efficiency in Health Care (IQWiG). Accessed May 28, 2020. https://www.informedhealth.org/how-does-our-sense-of-taste-work.2261.en.html.

68. Institute of Medicine (US) Committee on Use of Dietary Reference Intakes in Nutrition Labeling. 2003. "Dietary Reference Intakes: Guiding Principles for Nutrition Labeling and Fortification." Overview of Food Fortification in the United States and Canada. Washington (DC): National Academies Press

(US) 3. Accessed May 18, 2020. https://www.ncbi.nlm.nih.gov/books/NBK208880/.

69. International Agency for Research on Cancer. 2015. "Consumption of Red Meat and Processed Meat." IARC Working Group. IARC Monogr Eval Carcinog Risks Hum (in press) 114 (September): Lyon, 6–13. http://ucpvalencia.es/wp-content/uploads/2015/10/Lancet-Oncology.pdf.

70. Irwin, S. V., P. Fisher, E. Graham, A. Malek, and A. Robidoux. 2017. "Sulfites Inhibit the Growth of Four Species of Beneficial Gut Bacteria at Concentrations Regarded as Safe for Food." *PloS one* 12 (10): e0186629. https://doi.org/10.1371/journal.pone.0186629.

71. Jahns, L., W. Davis-Shaw, A. H. Lichtenstein, S. P. Murphy, Z. Conrad, and F. Nielsen. 2018. "The History and Future of Dietary Guidance in America." *Advances in Nutrition* 9 (2): 136–147. https://doi.org/10.1093/advances/nmx025.

72. Jamshed, H., R. A. Beyl, D. L. Della Manna, E. S. Yang, E. Ravussin, and C. M. Peterson. 2019. "Early Time-Restricted Feeding Improves 24-Hour Glucose Levels and Affects Markers of the Circadian Clock, Aging, and Autophagy in Humans." *Nutrients* 11 (6): 1234. https://doi.org/10.3390/nu11061234.

73. Jayawardene, W. P., M. R. Torabi, and D. K. Lohrman. 2016. "Exercise in Young Adulthood with Simultaneous and Future Changes in Fruit and Vegetable Intake." *Journal of the American College of Nutrition* 35 (1): 59–67. https://pubmed.ncbi.nlm.nih.gov/26251968/.

74. Jensen, T., M. F. Abdelmalek, S. Sullivan, K. J. Nadeau, M. Green, C. Roncal, T. Nakagawa, M. Kuwabara, Y. Sato, D. H. Kang, D. R. Tolan, L. G. Sanchez-Lozada, H. R. Rosen, M. A. Lanaspa, A. M. Diehl, and R. J. Johnson. 2018. "Fructose and Sugar: A Major Mediator of Non-alcoholic Fatty Liver Disease."

Journal of Hepatology 68 (5): 1063–1075. https://doi.org/10.1016/j.jhep.2018.01.019.

75. Jiang, Y., Y. Pan, P. R. Rhea, L. Tan, M. Gagea, L. Cohen, S. M. Fischer, and P. Yang. 2016. "A Sucrose-Enriched Diet Promotes Tumorigenesis in Mammary Gland in Part through the 12-Lipoxygenase Pathway." *Cancer Research* 76 (1): 24–29. https://doi.org/10.1158/0008-5472.CAN-14-3432.

76. Johnson, E. J. 2002. "The Role of Carotenoids in Human Health." *Nutr Clin Care Review* 5, no. 2 (March-April): 56–65. ncbi.nlm.nih.gov/pubmed/12134711.

77. Johnson, M. L., M. M. Robinson, and K. S. Nair. 2013. "Skeletal Muscle Aging and the Mitochondrion." *Trends in Endocrinology and Metabolism: TEM* 24 (5): 247–256. https://doi.org/10.1016/j.tem.2012.12.003.

78. Johnson, S. S., A. L. Paiva, C. O. Cummins, J. L. Johnson, S. J. Dyment, J. A. Wright, J. O. Prochaska, J. M. Prochaska, and K. Sherman. 2008. "Transtheoretical Model-Based Multiple Behavior Intervention for Weight Management: Effectiveness on a Population Basis." *Preventive Medicine* 46 (3): 238–246. https://doi.org/10.1016/j.ypmed.2007.09.010.

79. Kantor, E. D., C. D. Rehm, M. Du, E. White, and E. L. Giovannucci. 2016. "Trends in Dietary Supplement Use Among US Adults from 1999–2012." *JAMA* 316 (14): 1464–1474. https://doi.org/10.1001/jama.2016.14403.

80. Katafuchi, A., A. Sassa, N. Niimi, P. Grúz, H. Fujimoto, C. Masutani, F. Hanaoka, T. Ohta, and T. Nohmi. 2010. "Critical Amino Acids in Human DNA Polymerases η and κ Involved in Erroneous Incorporation of Oxidized Nucleotides," *Nucleic Acids Research* 38 (3): 859–867. https://doi.org/10.1093/nar/gkp1095.

81. Khoshnoud, M. J., A. Siavashpour, M. Bakhshizadeh, M. Rashedinia. 2018. "Effects of Sodium Benzoate, a Commonly Used Food Preservative, on Learning, Memory, and Oxidative Stress in Brain of Mice." *Journal of Biochemical and Molecular Toxicology*: 2 (2). https://doi.org/10.1002/jbt.22022.

82. Kiela, P. R., and F. K. Ghishan. 2016. "Physiology of Intestinal Absorption and Secretion." Best Practice & Research. *Clinical Gastroenterology* 30 (2): 145–159. https://www.ncbi.nlm.nih.gov/pmc/articles/PMC4956471/.

83. Kolb, B., R. Mychasiuk, A. Muhammad, Y. Li, D. O. Frost, and R. Gibb. 2012. "Experience and the Developing Prefrontal Cortex." Proceedings of the National Academy of Sciences of the United States of America. 109 (Suppl 2): 17186–17193. https://doi.org/10.1073/pnas.1121251109.

84. Koliaki, C., T. Spinos, M. Spinou, M. E. Brinia, D. Mitsopoulou, and N. Katsilambros. 2018. "Defining the Optimal Dietary Approach for Safe, Effective and Sustainable Weight Loss in Overweight and Obese Adults." *Healthcare* 6 (3): 73. https://doi.org/10.3390/healthcare6030073.

85. Koning, R. E. 1994. "Fruit Ripening." Plant Physiology Information. Accessed April 19, 2019. https://s8.lite.msu.edu/res/msu/botonl/b_online/library/koning/Plants_Human/fruitgrowripe.html.

86. Kyeong, S., J. Kim, D. J. Kim, H. E. Kim, and J. J. Kim. 2017. "Effects of Gratitude Meditation on Neural Network Functional Connectivity and Brain-Heart Coupling." *Scientific Reports* 7 (1): 5058. https://doi.org/10.1038/s41598-017-05520-9.

87. La Gorce, T. 2011. "The Tastemakers." *New Jersey Monthly*, January 17, 2011. https://njmonthly.com/articles/eat-drink/the-tastemakers/.

88. Lange, S. S., K. Takata, and R. D. Wood. 2011. "DNA Polymerases and Cancer." *Nature Reviews Cancer* 11 (2): 96–110. https://doi.org/10.1038/nrc2998.

89. Lattimer, J., and M. Haub. 2010. "Effects of Dietary Fiber and Its Components on Metabolic Health." *Nutrients* 2 (12): 1266–1289. https://doi.org/10.3390/nu2121266.

90. Lee, J. H., and H. S. Jun. 2019. "Role of Myokines in Regulating Skeletal Muscle Mass and Function." *Frontiers in Physiology* 10: 42. https://doi.org/10.3389/fphys.2019.00042.

91. Liauchonak, I., B. Qorri, F. Dawoud, Y. Riat, and M. R. Szewczuk. 2019. "Non-Nutritive Sweeteners and Their Implications on the Development of Metabolic Syndrome." *Nutrients* 11 (3): 644. https://doi.org/10.3390/nu11030644.

92. Lisle, D. J., and A. Goldhamer. 2006. *The Pleasure Trap: Mastering the Hidden Force That Undermines Health and Happiness.* Summertown, UK: Healthy Living.

93. Lloyd-Jones, D. M., P. B. Morris, C. M. Ballantyne, K. K. Birtcher, D. D. Daly, S. M. Depalma, M. B. Minissian, C. E. Orringer, and S. C. Smith. 2016. "ACC Expert Consensus Decision Pathway on the Role of Non-Statin Therapies for LDL-Cholesterol Lowering in the Management of Atherosclerotic Cardiovascular Disease Risk: A Report of the American College of Cardiology Task Force on Clinical Expert Consensus Documents." *Journal of the American College of Cardiology* 68 (1): 92–125. https://doi.org/10.1016/j.jacc.2016.03.519.

94. Lonnie, M., E. Hooker, J. M. Brunstrom, B. M. Corfe, M. A. Green, A. W. Watson, E. A. Williams, E. J. Stevenson, S. Penson, and A. M. Johnstone. 2018. "Protein for Life: Review of Optimal Protein Intake, Sustainable Dietary Sources and the Effect on Appetite in Ageing Adults." *Nutrients* 10 (3): 360. https://doi.org/10.3390/nu10030360.

95. Low M., M. Hayward, S. Appleyard, M. Rubinstein. 2003. "State-Dependent Modulation of Feeding Behavior by Proopiomelanocortin-Derived Beta-Endorphin." *Ann N Y Acad Sci*. 994 (1): 192–201. https://doi.org/10.1111/j.1749-6632.2003.tb03180.x.

96. Mäkinen, K. 2016. "Gastrointestinal Disturbances Associated with the Consumption of Sugar Alcohols with Special Consideration of Xylitol: Scientific Review and Instructions for Dentists and Other Health-Care Professionals." *International Journal of Dentistry*. 5967907. https://doi.org/10.1155/2016/5967907.

97. Maroulakis, E., and Y. Zervas. 1993. "Effects of Aerobic Exercise on Mood of Adult Women." *Perceptual and Motor Skills* 76 (3): 795–801. https://doi.org/10.2466/pms.1993.76.3.795.

98. May, P. 2017. "Vitamin B1 (Thiamine) Deficiency of This Causes Beriberi." University of Bristol. Accessed May 11, 2020. http://www.chm.bris.ac.uk/motm/vitaminB1/vitaminb1h.htm.

99. McEwen, B. S., and P. J. Gianaros. 2010. "Central Role of the Brain in Stress and Adaptation: Links to Socioeconomic Status, Health, and Disease." *Annals of the New York Academy of Sciences* 1186 (1): 190–222. https://doi.org/10.1111/j.1749-6632.2009.05331.x.

100. McEwen, B. S., J. M. Weiss, and L. S. Schwartz. 1968. "Selective Retention of Corticosterone by Limbic Structures in Rat Brain." *Nature* 220 (5170): 911–912. https://doi.org/10.1038/220911a0.

101. Meerman, R., and A. J. Brown. 2014. "When Somebody Loses Weight, Where Does the Fat Go?" *BMJ* (Clinical research ed.) 349: g7257. https://doi.org/10.1136/bmj.g7257.

102. Morbidity and Mortality Weekly Report (MMWR). 2004. "Spina Bifida and Anencephaly before and after Folic Acid Mandate." Accessed May 16, 2020. https://www.cdc.gov/mmwr/preview/mmwrhtml/mm5317a3.htm.

103. Murgia, C., and M. M. Adamski. 2017. "Translation of Nutritional Genomics into Nutrition Practice: The Next Step." *Nutrients* 9 (4): 366. https://doi.org/10.3390/nu9040366.

104. Murphy, G. 2003. "Mother's Diet Changes Pups' Colour." *Nature*. https://doi.org/10.1038/news030728-12.

105. Mutch, D. M., W. Wahli, and G. Williamson. 2005. "Nutrigenomics and Nutrigenetics: The Emerging Faces of Nutrition." *FASEB Journal* 19: 1602–1612. https://doi.org/10.1096/fj.05-3911rev.

106. National Center for Biotechnology Information. n.d. PubChem Database. Ethyl methylphenylglycidate, CID=650. Accessed May 17, 2020. https://pubchem.ncbi.nlm.nih.gov/compound/Ethyl-methylphenylglycidate.

107. National Center for Biotechnology Information. n.d. PubChem Database. Furaneol, CID=19309. Accessed May 17, 2020. https://pubchem.ncbi.nlm.nih.gov/compound/Furaneol.

108. National Center for Biotechnology Information (2022). PubChem Compound Summary for CID 19309, Furaneol. Retrieved August 17, 2022. https://pubchem.ncbi.nlm.nih.gov/compound/19309.

109. Navarro, S. L., F. Li, and J. W. Lampe. 2011. "Mechanisms of Action of Isothiocyanates in Cancer Chemoprevention: An Update." *Food and Function* 2 (10): 579–587. https://doi.org/10.1039/c1fo10114e.

110. Niaz, K., E. Zaplatic, and J. Spoor. 2018. "Extensive Use of Monosodium Glutamate: A Threat to Public Health?" *EXCLI Journal* 17: 273–278. https://doi.org/10.17179/excli2018-1092.

111. Nieman, D. C., and L. M. Wentz. 2019. "The Compelling Link between Physical Activity and the Body's Defense System." *Journal of Sport and Health Science* 8 (3): 201–217. https://doi.org/10.1016/j.jshs.2018.09.009.

112. Nix, E. 2018. "Who Invented Sliced Bread?" History.com. Accessed May 16, 2020. https://www.history.com/news/who-invented-sliced-bread.

113. NH DHHS-DPHS-Health Promotion in Motion. n.d. "How Much Sugar Do You Eat? You May Be Surprised!" Accessed May 25, 2020. https://www.studocu.com/en-ca/document/niagara-college-canada/sports-nutrition-practicum/sugar-lecture-notes-4/24239331.

114. Ochoa-Repáraz, J., and L. H. Kasper. 2016. "The Second Brain: Is the Gut Microbiota a Link between Obesity and Central Nervous System Disorders?" *Current Obesity Reports* 5 (1): 51–64. https://doi.org/10.1007/s13679-016-0191-1.

115. Olsen C. M. 2011. "Natural Rewards, Neuroplasticity, and Non-Drug Addictions." *Neuropharmacology* 61 (7): 1109–1122. https://doi.org/10.1016/j.neuropharm.2011.03.010.

116. Ou, C., S. Tsao, M. Lin, M. Yin. 2003. "Protective Action on Human LDL against Oxidation and Glycation by Four Organosulfur Compounds Derived from Garlic." *Lipids* 38: 219–224. https://doi.org/10.1007/s11745-003-1054-4.

117. Pandir, D. 2016. "DNA Damage in Human Germ Cell Exposed to Some Food Additives in Vitro." *Cytotechnology* 68 (4): 725–733. https://doi.org/10.1007/s10616-014-9824-y.

118. Papadopoulou, S. K. 2020. "Sarcopenia: A Contemporary Health Problem among Older Adult Populations." *Nutrients* 12 (5): 1293. https://doi.org/10.3390/nu12051293.

119. Patel, S. 2015. "Emerging Trends in Nutraceutical Applications of Whey Protein and Its Derivatives." *Journal of Food Science and Technology* 52 (11): 6847–6858. https://doi.org/10.1007/s13197-015-1894-0.

120. Phaniendra, A., D. B. Jestadi, and L. Periyasamy. 2015. "Free Radicals: Properties, Sources, Targets, and Their Implication in Various Diseases." *Indian Journal of Clinical Biochemistry* 30 (1): 11–26. https://doi.org/10.1007/s12291-014-0446-0.

121. Piercy, K. L., R. P. Troiano, R. M. Ballard, S. A. Carlson, J. E. Fulton, D. A. Galuska, S. M. George, and R. D. Olson, 2018. "The Physical Activity Guidelines for Americans." *JAMA* 320 (19): 2020–2028. https://doi.org/10.1001/jama.2018.14854.

122. Pignatelli, P., F. M. Pulcinelli, A. Celestini, L. Lenti, A. Ghiselli, P. P. Gazzaniga, and F. Violi. 2000. "The Flavonoids Quercetin and Catechin Synergistically Inhibit Platelet Function by Antagonizing the Intracellular Production of Hydrogen Peroxide." *American Journal of Clinical Nutrition* 72 (5): 1150–1155. https://doi.org/10.1093/ajcn/72.5.1150.

123. Pizzorno J. 2014. "Mitochondria-Fundamental to Life and Health." *Integrative Medicine* 13 (2): 8–15. https://www.ncbi.nlm.nih.gov/pmc/articles/PMC4684129/.

124. Prescott, S. L. 2017. "History of Medicine: Origin of the Term Microbiome and Why It Matters." *Human Microbiome Journal* 4: 24–25. https://dx.doi.org/10.1016/j.humic.2017.05.004.

125. Pressman, P., R. Roger Clemens, W. Hayes, and C. Reddy. 2017. "Food Additive Safety: A Review of Toxicologic and Regulatory Issues." *Toxicology Research and Application* 1: 1–22. sagepub.co.uk/journalsPermissions.nav. https://doi.org/10.1177/2397847317723572.

126. Raichle, M. E., and D. A. Gusnard. 2002. "Appraising the Brain's Energy Budget." *Proceedings of the National Academy of Sciences of the United States of America* 99 (16): 10237–10239. https://doi.org/10.1073/pnas.172399499.

127. Rakova, N., K. Kitada, K. Lerchl, A. Dahlmann, A. Birukov, S. Daub, C. Kopp, T. Pedchenko, Y. Zhang, L. Beck, B. Johannes, A. Marton, D. N. Müller, M. Rauh, F. C. Luft, and J. Titze. 2017. "Increased Salt Consumption Induces Body Water Conservation and Decreases Fluid Intake." *Journal of Clinical Investigation* 127 (5): 1932–1943. https://doi.org/10.1172/JCI88530.

128. Rao, P., R. Rodriguez, and S. Shoemaker. 2018. "Addressing the Sugar, Salt, and Fat Issue the Science of Food Way." *NPJ Science of Food* 2: 12. https://doi.org/10.1038/s41538-018-0020-x.

129. Rehman, I., N. Mahabadi, T. Sanvictores, and C. I. Rehman. 2020. "Classical Conditioning." In *StatPearls*. StatPearls Publishing, Treasure Island (FL). https://www.ncbi.nlm.nih.gov/books/NBK470326/.

130. Riebl, S. K., and B. M. Davy. 2013. "The Hydration Equation: Update on Water Balance and Cognitive Performance." *ACSM's Health and Fitness Journal* 17 (6): 21–28. https://doi.org/10.1249/FIT.0b013e3182a9570f.

131. Roberfroid, M. 1993. "Dietary Fiber, Insulin, and Oligofructose: A Review Comparing Their Physiological Effects." *Critical Reviews in Food Science and Nutrition* 33 (2): 103–148. https://www.tandfonline.com/doi/abs/10.1080/10408399309527616.

132. Rocha, J., J. Paxman, C. Dalton, E. Winter, and D. R. Broom. 2016. "Effects of a 12-week Aerobic Exercise Intervention on Eating Behaviour, Food Cravings, and 7-Day Energy Intake and Energy expenditure in Inactive Men." *Applied Physiology, Nutrition, and Metabolism* = Physiologie appliquee, nutrition et metabolisme 41 (11): 1129–1136. https://doi.org/10.1139/apnm-2016-0189.

133. Rolls, E. T. 2019. "Taste and Smell Processing in the Brain." *Handbook of Clinical Neurology* 164: 97–118. https://doi.org/10.1016/B978-0-444-63855-7.00007-1.

134. Roper, S. D., and N. Chaudhari. 2017. "Taste Buds: Cells, Signals and Synapses. Nature Reviews." *Neuroscience* 18 (8): 485–497. https://doi.org/10.1038/nrn.2017.68.

135. Sarafoleanu, C., C. Mella, M. Georgescu, and C. Perederco. 2009. "The Importance of the Olfactory Sense in the Human Behavior and Evolution." *Journal of Medicine and Life* 2 (2): 196–198. https://www.ncbi.nlm.nih.gov/pmc/articles/PMC3018978/.

136. Sarbani, G., J. Witta, J. Zhong, W. de Villiers, and E. Eckhardt. 2009. "Chylomicrons Promote Intestinal Absorption of Lipopolysaccharides." *J. Lipid Res* 50 (1): 90–97. https://doi.org/10.1194/jlr.M800156-JLR200.

137. Sender, R., S. Fuchs, and R. Milo. 2016. "Revised Estimates for the Number of Human and Bacteria Cells in the Body." *PLoS Biology* 14 (8): e1002533. https://doi.org/10.1371/journal.pbio.1002533.

138. Shouval, H. Z., S. S. Wang, and G. M. Wittenberg. 2010. "Spike Timing Dependent Plasticity: A Consequence of More Fundamental Learning Rules." *Frontiers in Computational Neuroscience* 4: 19. https://doi.org/10.3389/fncom.2010.00019.

139. Simopoulos, A. P. 2016. "An Increase in the Omega-6/Omega-3 Fatty Acid Ratio Increases the Risk for Obesity." *Nutrients* 8 (3): 128. https://doi.org/10.3390/nu8030128.

140. Singh, R. K., H. W. Chang, D. Yan, K. M. Lee, D. Ucmak, K. Wong, M. Abrouk, B. Farahnik, M. Nakamura, T. H. Zhu, T. Bhutani, and W. Liao. 2017. "Influence of Diet on the Gut Microbiome and Implications for Human Health." *Journal of Translational Medicine* 15 (1): 73. https://doi.org/10.1186/s12967-017-1175-y.

141. Springmann, M., M. Clark, and D. Mason-D'Croz, K. Wiebe, B. L. Bodirsky, L. Lassaletta, W. de Vries, S.J. Vermeulen, M.

Herrero, K.M. Carlson, M. Jonell, M. Troell, F. DeClerck. L.J. Gordon, R. Zurayk, P. Scarborough, M.Rayner, B. Loken, J. Fanzo, H. Charles J. Godfray, D. Tilman, J. Rockström & W. Willett. 2018. "Options for Keeping the Food System within Environmental Limits." *Nature* 562: 519–525. https://doi.org/10.1038/s41586-018-0594-0.

142. Stangl, D., and S. Thuret. 2009. "Impact of Diet on Adult Hippocampal Neurogenesis." *Genes and Nutrition* 4 (4): 271–282. https://doi.org/10.1007/s12263-009-0134-5.

143. Statista. 2020. "Food and Candy Advertising Spending in the United States from 2018 to 2020 (in Billion U.S. Dollars)." Statista Research Department. Accessed May 17, 2020. https://www.statista.com/statistics/497895/food-candy-ad-spend-usa/.

144. Stenkula, K.G., and C. Erlanson-Albertsson. 2018. "Adipose Cell Size: Importance in Health and Disease." *Am J Physiol Regul Integr Comp Physiol* 315: R284–R295. https://journals.physiology.org/doi/full/10.1152/ajpregu.00257.2017.

145. Stevens, L. J., J. R. Burgess, M. A. Stochelski, and T. Kuczek. 2013. "Amounts of Artificial Food Colors in Commonly Consumed Beverages and Potential Behavioral Implications for Consumption in Children." *Clin Pediatr (Phila)* 53 (2): 133–140. https://doi.org/10.1177/0009922813502849.

146. Stone, M., L. Martyn, and C. Weaver. 2016. "Potassium Intake, Bioavailability, Hypertension, and Glucose Control." *Nutrients* 8 (7): 444. https://doi.org/10.3390/nu8070444.

147. Taren, A. A., P. J. Gianaros, C. M. Greco, E. K. Lindsay, A. Fairgrieve, K. W. Brown, R. K. Rosen, J. L. Ferris, E. Julson, A. L. Marsland, and J. D. Creswell. 2017. "Mindfulness Meditation Training and Executive Control Network Resting State Functional Connectivity: A Randomized Controlled Trial."

Psychosomatic Medicine 79 (6): 674–683. https://doi.org/10.1097/PSY.0000000000000466.

148. Thau, L., and P. Singh. 2019. "Anatomy, Central Nervous System." In *StatPearls* [Internet]. Treasure Island, FL: StatPearls Publishing. https://www.ncbi.nlm.nih.gov/books/NBK542179/.

149. The Society of Flavor Chemists. n.d. "What Is the Difference between a Flavorist and a Flavor Chemist?" Accessed August 21, 2022. https://flavorchemists.com/about/faq/.

150. Thielecke, F., and A. P. Nugent. 2018. "Contaminants in Grain—A Major Risk for Whole Grain Safety?" *Nutrients* 10 (9): 1213. https://doi.org/10.3390/nu10091213.

151. Thomas, H. S. 2010. "Feeding Beef Cattle: Tips for a Healthy, Pasture-Based Diet." *Mother Earth News: The Original Guide to Living Wisely*. Accessed May 22, 2020. https://www.motherearthnews.com/homesteading-and-livestock/raising-cattle/feeding-beef-cattle-healthy-diet.

152. Tomassi, G., and V. Silano. 1986. "An Assessment of the Safety of Tocopherols as Food Additives." *Food and Chemical Toxicology*, an international journal published for the British Industrial Biological Research Association 24 (10–11): 1051–1061. https://doi.org/10.1016/0278-6915(86)90288-7.

153. Tosi, P., J. He, A. Lovegrove, I. Gonzáles-Thuillier, S. Penson, and P. R. Shewry. 2018. "Gradients in Compositions in the Starchy Endosperm of Wheat Have Implications for Milling and Processing." *Trends in Food Science and Technology* 82: 1–7. https://doi.org/10.1016/j.tifs.2018.09.027.

154. University of California - San Diego. 2020. "Vicious Circles: Ring-Shaped DNA Provides Cancer Cells with a Malignant Twist." *ScienceDaily*. Accessed April 21, 2020. https://www.sciencedaily.com/releases/2019/11/191120131347.htm.

155. U.S. Department of Agriculture. n.d. "Wheat Sector at a Glance." Accessed October 5, 2020. https://www.ers.usda.gov/topics/crops/wheat/wheat-sector-at-a-glance/.

156. U.S. Department of Health and Human Services and U.S. Department of Agriculture. 2015. *2015–2020 Dietary Guidelines for Americans.* 8th ed. http://health.gov/dietaryguidelines/2015/guidelines/.

157. U.S. Food and Drug Administration. 2016. "You May Be Surprised by How Much Salt You're Eating." Accessed May 25, 2020. https://www.fda.gov/consumers/consumer-updates/you-may-be-surprised-how-much-salt-youre-eating?source=govdelivery.

158. Veening, J. G., and H. P. Barendregt. 2015. "The Effects of Beta-Endorphin: State Change Modification." *Fluids and Barriers of the CNS* 12: 3. https://doi.org/10.1186/2045-8118-12-3.

159. Wang, G. J., N. D. Volkow, J. Logan, N. R. Pappas, C. T. Wong, W. Zhu, N. Netusil, and J. S. Fowler. 2001. "Brain Dopamine and Obesity." *Lancet* 357 (9253): 354–357. https://doi.org/10.1016/s0140-6736(00)03643-6.

160. Wang, Y. H., and H. R. Irving. 2011. "Developing a Model of Plant Hormone Interactions." *Plant Signaling and Behavior* 6 (4): 494–500. https://doi.org/10.4161/psb.6.4.14558.

161. Watts, M., and S. Watts. 2016. "From Quern to Computer: The History of Flour Milling. Roller Milling: A Gradual Takeover." *Mills Archive*, September 6, 2016: 10–15. https://new.millsarchive.org/2016/09/06/from-quern-to-computer-the-history-of-flour-milling/.

162. Weingärtner, O., M. Böhm, and U. Laufs. 2009. "Controversial Role of Plant Sterol Esters in the Management of Hypercholesterolaemia." *European Heart Journal* 30 (4): 404–409. https://doi.org/10.1093/eurheartj/ehn580.

163. Wikipedia. 2020. "Conrad Elvehjem." Last modified May 4, 2020. https://en.wikipedia.org/wiki/Conrad_Elvehjem#cite_note-4.

164. Wikipedia. n.d. "Western Pattern Diet." Accessed April 25, 2020. https://en.wikipedia.org/w/index.php?title=Western_pattern_dietandoldid=952319162.

165. Wiss, D. A., N. Avena, and P. Rada. 2018. "Sugar Addiction: From Evolution to Revolution." *Frontiers in Psychiatry* 9: 545. https://doi.org/10.3389/fpsyt.2018.00545.

166. Yang, T., J. Doherty, B. Zhao, A. J. Kinchla, J. M. Clark, and L. He. 2017. "Effectiveness of Commercial and Homemade Washing Agents in Removing Pesticide Residues on and in Apples." *Journal of Agricultural and Food Chemistry* 65 (44): 9744–9752. https://doi.org/10.1021/acs.jafc.7b03118.

167. Yang, W., and P. Hu. 2018. "Skeletal Muscle Regeneration Is Modulated by Inflammation." *Journal of Orthopaedic Translation* 13: 25–32. https://doi.org/10.1016/j.jot.2018.01.002.

168. Yuan, P., and N. Raz. 2014. "Prefrontal Cortex and Executive Functions in Healthy Adults: A Meta-Analysis of Structural Neuroimaging Studies." *Neuroscience and Biobehavioral Reviews* 42: 180–192. https://doi.org/10.1016/j.neubiorev.2014.02.005.

169. Zeisel, S. H., & da Costa, K. A. (2009). Choline: an essential nutrient for public health. *Nutrition reviews*, 67(11), 615–623. https://doi.org/10.1111/j.1753-4887.2009.00246.x.

170. Zhao, Z., Q. Feng, Z. Yin, J. Shuang, B. Bai, P. Yu, M. Guo, and Q. Zhao. 2017. "Red and Processed Meat Consumption and Colorectal Cancer Risk: A Systematic Review and Meta-Analysis." *Oncotarget* 8 (47): 83306–83314. https://doi.org/10.18632/oncotarget.20667.

171. Zia, A., H. U. Siddiqui, H. Mohiuddin, and S. Gul. 2018. "Leveling-Off of Declining Trend of Cardiovascular Disease-Related Mortality in the USA: The Challenge to Rein in Obesity and Diabetes Epidemic." *Cardiovascular Endocrinology and Metabolism* 7 (2): 54–55. https://doi.org/10.1097/XCE.0000000000000146.

Made in the USA
Las Vegas, NV
26 December 2022